Desperate Rants
and
Magic Pants
Our fertility story

ABOUT THE BOOK

"Andrea's book is a must for anyone going through fertility issues. It's a reminder that you are not alone and sharing our stories with each other really can help to normalise and comfort in what can be a lonely time."

– **Gabby Logan, BBC sports presenter**

"Anyone navigating this hard journey has just found the warmest and most honest of companions in Andrea, who has brought all of her journalistic skills to the most personal of subjects."

– **Julie Etchingham, ITV News at Ten anchor**

"Andrea writes with such honesty and sensitivity about a subject so often unspoken of. Her enthusiasm as a journalist to tackle taboo subjects in a relatable and accessible way is truly refreshing."

– **Jason Watkins, actor**

"Going through fertility struggles can feel very isolating – the uncertainties and range of emotions are tough to navigate. The more we talk about it openly, the better."

– **Izzy Judd, violinist, author, podcast host & wife of *Strictly* winner Harry Judd**

"Andrea Byrne eloquently, emotionally and bravely relates her and her husband Lee's fertility story. This is a book which will be a source of strength and company for anyone grappling with infertility."

– **Sharon Martin, Fertility Network UK**

Desperate Rants and *Magic Pants*

Our fertility story

Andrea Byrne

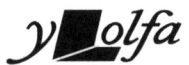

For my mum.
For supporting me unfailingly in my struggle to become a mum. The best listener of desperate rants I am ever likely to know.

Please be aware that there are references to baby loss and stillbirth in this book, which some may find distressing.

All information was correct as far as the author and the publishers were able to verify at the time of going to press (or at time of recording, in the podcast section).

First impression: 2024

© Copyright Andrea Byrne and Y Lolfa Cyf., 2024

The contents of this book are subject to copyright, and may not be reproduced by any means, mechanical or electronic, without the prior, written consent of the publishers.

The publishers wish to acknowledge
the support of the Books Council of Wales.

Cover design: Sion Ilar
Front cover image: Gemma Griffiths Photography
All other images © Andrea & Lee Byrne, unless otherwise stated

ISBN: 978-1-912631-51-3

Published and printed in Wales
on paper from well-maintained forests by
Y Lolfa Cyf., Talybont, Ceredigion SY24 5HE
website www.ylolfa.com
e-mail ylolfa@ylolfa.com
tel 01970 832 304

Contents

Foreword by Lee Byrne	7
Introduction	12
Prologue: Beginning of the end	16
1. Touch. Pause. Engage.	24
2. The infertility vortex	44
3. *Incroyable*	62
4. Rugby full-time, IVF half-time	81
5. Dying to hope	100
6. The American Dream	113
7. The club	127
8. Pip	133
Epilogue	145
Making Babies podcast stories	
Clare Nasir: On fibroids and fertility	151
Geoff Norcott: On stillbirth and men's mental health	160
Ria & Fern Burrage-Male: On IVF and sperm donation for same-sex couples	169
Kevin & Nicci Button: On male infertility	179
Danielle Beattie: On recurrent miscarriage	186
Stephen Ashe & Teresa Cootes: On surrogacy in the UK	191
Gabby Logan: Reflecting on fertility treatment	201
Glossary of technical terms	212
Acknowledgements	220

Foreword

by Lee Byrne

(long-suffering husband of a tenacious journalist)

As a disclaimer to whatever else I might write here – and to avoid that stern newsreader look she delivers so well when I'm in trouble – I love my wife very much and I have a huge amount of respect for what she does, and as a consequence what drives her.

But, blimey, it's pretty exhausting sometimes having a wife who's a journalist through and through, who's intent on righting wrongs, trying to create change and telling stories which might make those differences.

It's a discomfort that's magnified when you combine it with me, an intensely private person. Whilst I used to get an immense thrill from scoring a try in front of thousands of fans in a rugby stadium, the media spotlight isn't really for me. Though I've stepped into it on occasion during my sporting career, I'm very happy to quickly step back out.

When we were going through fertility treatment, I was particularly adamant that we shouldn't talk about it publicly – maybe because of my general nature or maybe because men just seem more inclined not to talk about anything personal. Fortunately, Andrea and I agreed on that. We both told only a very small circle of people we could call upon for support if we needed it. We didn't tell anyone at work, except those that had to know if we needed to be at a clinic. We kept it to ourselves. It had the plus of avoiding endless questions, yes, but also the minus of then making it a very isolating first few years as a newly married couple.

After the first three or four years, we both shared with a few more people. Largely because people do just seem to keep on asking when you're going to have children. Not *if*, but *when*. So I did say something to a few of the boys, in terms of letting people know we were trying, just to try to shut the conversation down for my own sanity.

The last thing I felt we needed was any kind of intrusion into the full degree of what was happening to us. I know I had it fairly easy on the physical side of things. It was Andrea going through all the tests, drugs, experiments, operations and more tests. With IVF, especially when the issue is more concerned with the woman, the guy's side is fairly minor on a practical level. We have to do *the thing* to produce the sample. Need I say more?

But Andrea's appointments, injections, treatments and tablets went on and on. And on top of that, we were both struggling emotionally. My thoughts would go off on tangents, wondering if a knock down below in rugby might have made some kind of difference to what I was producing, and maybe they just didn't know. It sounds crazy, because all the tests seemed fine, but your mind goes down strange paths. In the very same period I also lost one of my best friends – the All Black Jerry Collins. I was dealing with a lot.

Andrea was also finding it hard emotionally. She found it almost impossible to front up to family events like christenings, and even Christmas ended up being a painful reminder of what we didn't have.

Foreword

I found that less of a burden, but it was still hard to be fully engaged at an event or in a moment. It seemed like a front. And pretending we were OK was exhausting, and taking its toll behind closed doors, for sure. There were many times we felt at breaking point.

I say all this because from my point of view, the situation was hard enough to deal with in private: why would anyone want to make themselves so vulnerable as to share it all publicly if they didn't have to?

Well, after Jemima came along, this is exactly what Andrea wanted to do. Some good friends of ours, fellow newsreaders Hannah and Lewis Vaughan Jones, had shared their story of IVF as they went along. They'd written news articles and posted YouTube videos about the medical procedures. Andrea felt in awe of them having the strength to do this while they were in the midst of the storm. And I know every time she saw anyone talking about their fertility struggles on TV, she would get so emotional as it was such a relief to not feel so alone. Someone was there on national telly, saying, "This is bloody hard and I know no one talks about it, but people are here going through the same thing and there is hope." As a journalist, Andrea wanted to play her part in that. She wanted to normalise the conversation to help anyone on this wretched journey feel less alone in that storm.

Soon after having Jemima, I knew what was building. I knew she wanted to talk about it. She felt she owed it to others. By this point, I had started talking to a few more of the rugby boys about it. I'd mention IVF and several of them said they'd been through it. And I started to feel maybe this wasn't a shameful thing to keep under wraps.

More and more, I'd discover teammates or coaches who'd travelled the same road. I even began to use it more as a conversation starter, rather than a conversation stopper. If someone asked if we had children, or the next question: "Are you going to have any more?", I'd say, "It took us long enough to have the first one," and briefly explain the story.

I think aside from Andrea's need to scratch the storytelling itch to help others, her thinking was also similar to mine. She'd rather be in control of the narrative than leaving everyone to make up their own.

She tentatively contacted a trusted journalist friend of hers, Liz Perkins, from the print media in Wales, and asked if she'd be interested in writing something. I went along with it, although somewhat begrudgingly, because I did also believe that it could help other men if people talked about it more.

From there, Andrea wanted to do more to get the message out that we all need to chat about fertility and infertility as an everyday conversation, whether that be in the office, at a networking event, at the gym or down the pub.

Why was I not surprised that when we went into a global pandemic and were in lockdown, she created, produced and hosted her own podcast, talking to guests and looking at all aspects of infertility? It went into a second series, with her interviewing a variety of celebrities, some of whose stories you'll find in this book. I have one determined wife!

The book has been a labour of love. And whilst, if I'm honest, it's not something I would have done, I did believe in her reasons for doing it. Those reasons were

Foreword

only reinforced over and over again when I did some sort of social media post in relation to it – I would receive dozens of comments on social media from men going through fertility treatment, who felt that little bit less isolated when they heard my story.

Last but not least – and this is actually really important – it's not just for other couples having fertility issues. It's for family members, friends and colleagues who want to really understand what's happening in someone's world at this turbulent time. I think there's a perception that IVF is a miracle solution – a one-stop shop to get a baby if you're having issues. There's a bit of medicine involved and there you go: family made. But it's so much more complex than that in reality. By knowing what this experience can be like, hopefully others can react with empathy and say the right things – or at least not say the wrong things (of which there are many!).

Lee Byrne
September 2024

Introduction

DURING THE CORONAVIRUS pandemic, the idea emerged of creating and hosting a podcast. There were a lot of topics I could have chosen for a podcast, many of which would probably have been far less niche and, ultimately, attracted bigger audiences. But I really wanted to try to reach people who needed to feel included in a conversation – and there weren't a great deal of conversations about fertility going on in any form of media. And so I took a deep breath and created *Making Babies: A Fertility Podcast* (thanks to Andrew Wilson at Cloud Nine Management for the name!). This was a big step, because my husband Lee and I had been quite private about our story for a long time and creating a platform for other people to talk would inevitably mean a little bit more sharing on our part.

With the subject matter being so delicate and intimate, it seemed appropriate that the podcast was just me and a computer at a desk in my house – and that's the way it's always remained. When it all started, I was still working as a broadcaster throughout the lockdowns but with any social life a distant dream for us all, I spent my spare time learning how to use Zoom, how to edit audio effectively (trying to dig out the memories of my days in radio), how to send it where it needed to go and finding out which production apps to use to promote it effectively on social media. My thanks to the wonderful Abi, who helped me

Introduction

out with the techy issue of actually getting the podcast on the right platforms, which seemed to need a degree in itself – I'd taught myself a lot about podcast production by this stage, but that bit proved slightly too much for my brain to handle.

In October 2020, the first episode of the first series began with two brilliant guests and a conversation about the tips and tricks which can mentally and emotionally help you and others navigate fertility issues. Thank you to Fertility Network UK, which supported me in getting this off the ground and participated in the inaugural episode, and thanks to counsellor Wendy Martin too. We discussed so much of the stuff I'd have wanted to hear if it had been me just starting out on this muddle of a journey – not least the things not to say to people! I'm not sure if it was more cathartic for me or the listeners – or maybe it was doing both jobs, which was a bonus.

Once I was up and running, I was finding people were really keen to come on and talk about different aspects of the fertility conversation, and the first series turned into a bit of a guide on different specialist areas. We discussed miscarriage, surrogacy, male infertility, and holistic alternatives which might support medical treatments. Thank you to all those who took the time to participate in Series 1. The number of messages I received and the positive feedback from people I had never met was truly humbling. It felt as if *Making Babies* was really making a difference.

I decided to put a slightly different twist on it for the second series as I realised that there were a fair few celebrities who had been brave enough to talk about their struggles with conceiving and I realised this could be really inspiring. Whether I could pull it off was another matter entirely, but I had to have faith.

I began by approaching fellow female broadcaster and fellow rugby player's wife, the phenomenal Gabby Logan. Married to Kenny Logan, I was hopeful that the playing links with my husband Lee might just help sway Gabby to come on the show. She agreed and that set off a series of well-known guests, such as comedian Geoff Norcott, former *Love Island* star Jessica Hayes, author Izzy Judd (wife of McFly's Harry Judd), weather presenter Clare Nasir, newsreaders Hannah and Lewis Vaughan Jones and former Wales Hockey international Ria Burrage-Male.

As I mentioned, it evolved in such a way that the podcast became an outlet for me to start tentatively telling snippets of our story too. I don't think at that stage I was ready to write it all down, but *Making Babies* provided me with a way of talking about it in a journalistic interview style that would raise awareness and help others, but not be focused on our experiences alone.

Gradually, though, I knew I wanted to say more. The podcast reception gave me confidence to make a pitch for the book. I knew now there was an audience who needed these stories to help with their own. I broached it with Lee, who by this point I think had also accepted that we were helping people by sharing, and with his blessing I set about trying to make it happen.

That idea of a book became *this* book – which in the end has also been able to feature some of the many *Making Babies* guest stories: something that is really important to me in *Desperate Rants and Magic Pants*. It means I've been able to talk about what we went through, but also to

Introduction

represent all sorts of other experiences along the fertility spectrum. I know we won't have touched on everyone's, but I'm so happy that the book includes a representation of so many people's stories from the podcast. Each account that you'll read in the section near the end of the book is taken from a podcast conversation.

I am very proud of the podcast and also incredibly proud – considering the emotion involved – that I've been able to write our story down in some sort of coherent fashion. I didn't write this for sympathy, or for a whinge or a moan (although it has been cathartic to set it down with a purpose). Firstly, I wrote it to try to be a source of strength and company for people grappling with infertility. I hope I've achieved this. Secondly, I wrote it to help foster better awareness in those who are close to anyone struggling to start a family. It can be difficult to know how to open up the conversation. Well, maybe this book can help.

Every journey to a child is different and unique. I hope you find something that *you* can relate to in this book. You'll find the fertility story of me and my husband (who you've met in the Foreword) first, and later you'll find the podcast accounts.

If you'd like to see more from my work on fertility, my TedX talk *Fertility and The Forgotten Sex* and my Royal Television Award-winning documentary *Miscarriage: The Hidden Loss* are both available online. Thank you for your support.

Andrea Byrne

15

Prologue

Beginning of the end

It was Monday 21 May, 2018. This date I know, because it was the beginning of the end.

I'm in the dressing room at the ITV studios in Cardiff, getting ready for tonight's live news programme at 6 p.m. In the newsrooms outside of London, we do our own make-up and – although it may sound strange to my fellow presenters – I wouldn't have it any other way. For me, it provides a few minutes of quiet time alone to gather my thoughts, before we go into a routine of rehearsals and pre-recorded promotions and interviews, which run at quite a pace as we hurtle towards 'on-air' at 6 p.m. Whilst most people are heading home, winding down, preparing food and catching up on the evening headlines, for newsrooms, it's peak time.

In California, it is approaching 9 a.m. In the sunshine state they are just arriving for work. Lee and I have recently been having fertility treatment at a clinic in San Diego. As the clinicians fire up their computers and check in with the laboratory results overnight, they then go on to update their patients, usually via email. The emails come to me, partly due to Lee's dyslexia, and partly because I am desperate to feel like I am in control of something when actually, of course, by the very nature of infertility, I am in control of nothing.

Prologue: Beginning of the end

Six days ago, Linda from the lab team emailed to tell me how many embryos had survived of the ones we had produced during our in vitro fertilisation (IVF) cycle with them. Her email dropped in my inbox whilst we were on air. I saw it during the post-programme debrief, digesting the information whilst attempting to coherently contribute to a debate about the news show's content from that night. Linda's note ended by telling us that we would have the next results we were awaiting in 10 days' time.

The next results, we both know, are crucial. They will determine our future like no other results over the last six years.

Since we married in 2012, we'd had no success trying to conceive and we'd become unfortunate veterans of the fertility game. We'd endured multiple treatments in varying forms, both traditional and experimental. Our journey had taken us to clinics in Cardiff, London and France. The latter saw me taking an unpaid year-long sabbatical to join Lee in a city called Clermont-Ferrand, where he was playing professional rugby for three years.

Our medical motivation for my leave of absence was unknown to most people and I became the envy of my colleagues, who imagined me lucky enough to be able to indulge myself in a 12-month life-enriching continental experience. In reality, I was spending most of my time at hospital appointments being scanned, operated on, pumped full of hormone-altering drugs and navigating the intricacies of French infertility vocab. Although of course I knew we were still fortunate for me to be able to take the year away from work at all.

The experience at every clinic which treated us had followed a similar pattern. Perhaps there might be a small change in protocol and an experimental drug would be thrown into the treatment cycle, but the outcome was always the same: failure.

On some occasions, Lee's sperm did fertilise a good number of my eggs in the lab and we ended up with a decent number of embryos. But there was no pregnancy. On other occasions, we used embryos frozen from a previous cycle, but the treatment often barely got started before being cancelled. Once, from one of these cycles, there *may* have been a pregnancy. Possibly what's known as a chemical one, which is really a crude term for it being too early to tell if anything really happened or not. But that, too, came to nothing. On another occasion, there definitely was a pregnancy. But that ended in early miscarriage.

The failure was always put down to one thing, on repeat. It was never, we were told, the quality or quantity of the embryos we were producing, which is so often the issue for couples. According to what could be seen under a microscope, they were OK. For us, it was always the fragility and thinness of my womb lining that was the problem. Fun fertility fact for you: for an embryo to 'stick' in the womb and start a pregnancy, a woman's womb lining should ideally be at least 8 mm thick. Well, mine was often only edging past 3 mm. And so, eventually, each doctor would conclude the same thing. I had what seemed to be an unfixable rare genetic defect. We had to accept I probably couldn't carry a child.

So we had changed course. Quite drastically. To California. In the States, we were doing something

Prologue: Beginning of the end

vastly different. And to do it, we needed to know whether our embryos really *were* OK, or if they had hidden chromosomal defects – issues that apparently couldn't even be seen on first inspection in the lab.

Why? Because with our new plan, it would not be the thickness of my womb lining that mattered.

Why? Because I wouldn't be the one carrying our baby.

Why? Because the reason we had travelled to America was to find a surrogate mother.

That's right. Deep breath. Big move. Another woman – a woman we'd not yet met – would be 'hosting' our embryo and growing our child. Because I couldn't.

But hold on. Pause a moment. I think I may have just made the transition from IVF treatment to surrogacy sound like an easy one. But at the time when we were trying to become parents, it was anything but:

1. Commercial surrogacy was (and at time of writing still is) illegal in the UK, although you can pay a friend on an expenses-only basis.
2. *But* this was only possible if you knew a friend or relative willing to do it. Otherwise, you needed to sign up to a non-profit matching agency.
3. *But*, at that time there was a shortage of surrogates coming forward through this means, and non-profit agencies which pair 'intended parents' (me and Lee) with a surrogate had stopped taking on new clients. Fortunately, this situation has now massively improved, but for us, the other option to consider was going abroad to somewhere with a manageable price tag and reasonably close to home. Somewhere like Eastern Europe.
4. *But* Eastern Europe, despite being reasonably-priced, lacked a sufficiently developed bureaucratic and legal

19

framework to ensure safe and efficient passage of parents and babies with passports back to the UK post-delivery. America, however, has well-developed and sound legislation in place.
5. *But* American surrogacy comes at a cost which is insurmountable for most people.

There you go. I think that sums it up pretty well for now. Not an easy move to make.

However, despite having already spent thousands of pounds on treatment, we did register for surrogacy in America. In the end, the decision to pursue a new life in a new way came from another life being taken far too soon. My father passed away suddenly in early 2017. He knew of our desperation to have a family and, to me, it seemed undeniably appropriate that we should use his legacy to enable us to pursue the possibility of creating his grandchild.

So we had written our letters and sent our photographs to a surrogacy agency in the States, hoping that a surrogate mum somewhere on the West Coast would go through the files, like us and pick us. It's a complex process to get there, though. Surrogacy isn't widely talked about, so let me give you a snapshot of how it all works.

The in vitro fertilisation (IVF) side of things is largely the same. First, I have injections of hormones during the first half of my menstrual cycle to stimulate my ovaries to produce an unnatural number of eggs that month (usually a woman produces one egg per month in her menstrual cycle).

Alongside these injections, I have a series of ultrasound scans on my ovaries to tell the doctors when the optimum time is to operate in order to remove – 'harvest' – the

Prologue: Beginning of the end

eggs. Then the eggs are fertilised with Lee's sperm, or sometimes one sperm is directly injected into each egg. Some will survive and create embryos which could create babies, others will not. The embryos which are created are left to develop in the lab. Again, some will survive, others will not. A few days later, the surviving embryos – if they look to be good quality – are frozen. At a later date, one or maybe more will be thawed and transferred to the womb of the surrogate mother.

As I'm sitting in the dressing room on 21 May 2018, what we already know from Linda in California is that from our cycle in San Diego we have ended up with three 'good-looking' embryos, considered suitable for use. Not a bad result. Up until now, the test and results process is all fairly familiar to us from previous cycles. But there's one more hurdle to overcome with the embryos. And this part is all new.

Following their survival, our three embryos were sent for what's known as preimplantation genetic screening (PGS) – which has actually since become a controversial procedure. In America, this was an obligatory part of the surrogacy process, and it seemed to make sense. It's meant to give everyone the least chance of traumatic failure and the best chance of success. And it's even more important as a woman gets older and her embryos become more vulnerable to being faulty. The screening looks at the chromosomes of each embryo. A normal embryo will have a normal number of chromosomes. 'Normal' means a higher chance of implantation and a lower chance of miscarriage and/or birth defects.

It is these results we are waiting on. If one embryo tests as chromosomally normal, it's the beginning of our surrogacy journey in earnest. Without a normal embryo from this testing, it's game over.

I'm not expecting any news that particular day – I thought it was too soon. So I'm hot-brushing my hair; I'm applying my lipliner; I'm tweeting about what we have coming up on the programme; I'm running through my interview topics; and I'm listening to other broadcasters' headlines on the radio.

I can't remember why now, but I check my email. Maybe in those days I still had pop-up notifications on. Or maybe we were awaiting some last-minute confirmation on details of a story. Whatever the reason, four days earlier than expected, a new email from San Diego is there. I start to panic and sweat. My stomach begins to churn. My heart rate soars. None of these feelings are new. In fact, they have become my normal. I've lived with anxiety for a long time now. But today, the stakes are at their highest.

With all things fertility, where you hardly dare to be optimistic for fear of having your hopes crushed, I have in fact been cautiously upbeat about the PGS test results. My reasoning? We've taken a huge decision to go down the route of surrogacy. Huge emotionally, huge physically and huge financially. I suppose I feel we deserve a break. I feel we deserve these results for letting go of the hopes of my own pregnancy and accepting a different way forward.

I open the email.

NO embryos have tested as 'normal'. Not one single embryo. Zero. After hoping and planning for months, injecting drugs again for weeks and spending tens of thousands of pounds, the result is failure. Again.

Prologue: Beginning of the end

In a matter of seconds, darkness consumes the sliver of light I've dared to let in. I am empty and nauseous at the same time. A familiar feeling. I know that even if I don't spiral into emotional disaster right now, it is only a matter of time. Quickly the 'what ifs' I have worked so hard to banish come scurrying out from the nooks and crannies of my mind.

"What if the embryos all fail? What is our future?"

"What if the embryos all fail? Will Lee even want to stay with me?"

"What if the embryos all fail? What's the point in anything anymore?"

This feels like the end.

I sit, motionless. My painted face is illuminated by a surround of spotlights in the mirror. It's a metaphor for what life has become. A continuous masking of our painful reality from the world. And then, as on so many other occasions, I look at my tear-streaked reflection in the mirror, patch up the damaged foundation, breathe deeply, walk out of the dressing room, put on a smile and walk through a busy newsroom, and on to the set.

"Good evening. I'm Andrea Byrne. Welcome to the programme."

There is no other way forward now. I can't fix this. I can't make things work. This is the end, I tell myself.

In fact, in so many ways, it is a new beginning.

But, first, as the song goes – let's start at the *very* beginning. It's a very good place to start.

23

Chapter 1

Touch. Pause. Engage.

I WAS 33 when Lee and I married. It was New Year's Day 2012. 01.01.12. I know many people might consider 33 late to first marry, but it never seemed that way to me. I think for a woman that depends on a lot of different influences and where life ends up taking you.

Firstly, I always had in mind that my mum did not fall pregnant with me until she was 33 and she had me when she was 34. Rightly or wrongly, it seemed the natural thing for me to measure my marriage and childbearing goals against. Back in the Seventies, she told me she was medically considered a 'geriatric' mother by midwives. And, in my mind, decades had passed since then and society's attitudes had much progressed. And so marrying – and looking to fall pregnant – at 33 still felt young-ish. I still felt I had plenty of time.

Secondly, and more importantly, I also had in mind that it was first and foremost about finding the right person. I had opportunities to marry and 'settle down' earlier, but I bailed. As much as I was in love at the time, in the end circumstances meant it didn't work. It was not meant to be. I hope this second point also corrects assumptions (and there have been many) that the delay was due to my career aspirations. Yes, my career had been going well and I was on an upwards trajectory, gaining promotions and opportunities. But it was never a conscious driving factor in delaying other life decisions. I think women can be all too unfairly judged on this.

I do sometimes consider that it is just in my nature somehow, though, to leave milestones a little later in life. Perhaps until I'm really sure. I recently completed one of those surveys used in business to tell you what type of personality you are to work with. I came up, first and foremost, as a precisionist. I put off doing things until I am certain I can proceed and secure the best result. Great for accuracy and attention to detail, but inevitably that can often mean I'm late to the party.

When I look back on the four decades (plus!) I have been on this planet, I have been late to the party a lot. OK, yes – often quite literally too! My husband would wholeheartedly agree with this in terms of my timekeeping for nearly every event – bar the on-air countdown to a news programme. For that, I always make it. Otherwise, he claims, I faff. I won't leave the house until I have checked every single thing it's possible to check. And the same can be applied to life events. If given the chance, with any sort of important decision or test, he's right: I do faff. Too fearful to risk getting it wrong or failing. Precision. Is. Key. Right?

It may have all been destined from birth. I was born in October, for starters, which means I was one of the eldest in my school year. This means you are always on the back foot, in a way. I went to middle school at almost 10 instead of just turned 9; I sat my GCSEs at nearly 17 instead of just turned 16; my A-levels at nearly 19 instead of just turned 18. Well – you get my drift. Granted, it wasn't a huge chasm at that age and actually it should have had its perks, particularly in terms of something like learning to drive. As I was one of the eldest in the year, I was one of the first to take lessons. The only problem was, the precisionist in me took so long having lessons that by the time I was ready to take the test, a lot of my peers had caught up with me, if not overtaken (excuse the pun!).

Overall, it didn't bother me that much at the time, but as I started to make decisions, I exacerbated the effect. Firstly, I took a gap year and travelled to Bali, Australia and New Zealand, which made me even later to university. Then after my three-year degree I did a year's postgraduate diploma in Broadcast Journalism, which delayed me getting a job for a further year. In fact, when I did start in my first full-time job in journalism, I was a few months shy of 24! My sister, conversely, has an August birthday so was possibly the youngest in her year. She took no gap year and did a standard three-year undergrad degree. She was in the workplace when she turned 21. She was married at 24 and had her first child four years later. I would always be playing catch-up.

It wasn't just my educational choices that slowed everything down a pace or two. My agonising precision affected my relationships too. Despite several long-term relationships of three years, five years and six years, serial monogamy seemed to be my thing. Something like 'practice makes perfect', I guess I thought. It wasn't until I was 32 years old that I met my husband. Then, largely thanks to *his* personality type and not mine, we were engaged within five months and married in another nine. I had seemingly met my antithesis in terms of impulsivity – a risk-taker who waits for nothing and no

1. Touch. Pause. Engage.

one. But they do say opposites attract. And little did we know it, but the path to that attraction actually began four years earlier.

In January 2008, I moved to Wales after being offered my dream job as the main anchor on a flagship news programme. I'd been a producer, editor and reporter in various guises for eight years on radio and on TV and this move west, from ITV regional news in the south of England to national news in Wales, was my biggest break so far.

I was determined to settle into Welsh life quickly and part of that was discovering what mattered to Wales. If you're Welsh yourself, if you've ever visited for any length of time, or in fact if you know anyone who is Welsh, then you'll know that rugby union is a religion here. And in January, in Wales, you are guaranteed headlines of one kind: an impassioned build-up to and analysis of Six Nations rugby. The Six Nations tournament sees Northern hemisphere teams Wales, England, Ireland, Scotland, France and Italy competing to be champions and perhaps also Grand Slam-winners – a prize that's awarded to any team who beat every other team they play that year.

During my first week in the newsroom, I quickly realised that knowing the stars of the Welsh squad was as important as knowing the politicians in the Welsh cabinet. I took the double-page team photograph from the centre of the *Western Mail* newspaper and I stuck it up by my desk, with each player's name written by their headshot. This was just as much a 'new girl' exercise in public relations, I suppose, as it was a serious educational tool. I didn't only learn names, but the poster became a

27

talking point – and very quickly I also found out that the regional team making the biggest impact in the Wales squad that year was a club called the Ospreys.

The Ospreys of the Noughties gained the tag 'Galacticos' after the club spent big on International names. The squad line-up boasted several British Lions (the highest level a player can reach in British and Irish rugby) and two All Blacks. The roll-call included the late Jerry Collins, Filo Tiatia, Tommy Bowe, Lee Byrne, Mike Philips, Shane Williams, James Hook and Gavin Henson. So it was no surprise that the so-called Galacticos dominated the national squad that year: 13 of the Wales squad for the Six Nations were Galacticos.

The talk was about one group of players in particular, who had emerged with the nickname 'The Fab Four'. And so, being the men of the moment, it was these players I learnt of first. Shane Williams – winger and Wales' top try scorer, Mike Philips – scrum half, James Hook – fly half, and full back Lee Byrne.

There seemed no escaping Lee Byrne. Every night we would go into the studio at around 5.30 p.m. to record the promotions for the programme that night. And most nights at that time there was an advert running for a gold-trading company called Cash for Gold. It featured none other than Mr Byrne and, most evenings, it would play out just before we went live at 6 p.m. It involved him in his trunks, diving into a swimming pool and then surfacing clutching a fistful of gold chains, necklaces and other jewellery. I don't remember the script. I'm guessing that could be because we often only saw the pictures without audio, if we were practising lines and connecting with reporters live on location. Or it might be

1. Touch. Pause. Engage.

because the image distracted from the words! Either way, it was an ad that seemed to run on repeat at that time of the day. Another piece of subliminal Lee brainwashing.

As it turned out, the nation didn't need a Cash for Gold ad for Lee Byrne and his 2008 colleagues to become household names. Wales won the tournament that year and with it the Triple Crown (beating England, Scotland and Ireland) and the Grand Slam (beating all teams in the competition). But perhaps bigger than any trophy, they had beaten England on their own turf, at the hallowed Twickenham. One for the record books, as they say. At the time, Wales hadn't won there in two decades. And one of Wales' two try scorers that day was full back Lee Byrne. The moment is captured in a still photograph as he touches down in the foreground, leaving England's legendary Jonny Wilkinson for dust in the background. To this day, it has pride of place in our house.

The following week on the news, I remember I was presenting and the Six Nations trophy was brought into the studio for me and my co-presenter Jonathan Hill to hold in the opening title sequence. I'm not sure that, as a recent migrant to Wales, I fully understood in those days what it meant to the nation, if I'm honest. Now, nearly twenty years in Wales, I know a lot more of how the fortunes of Welsh rugby had played out in the preceding decades, appreciate that Wales had been through some dark times in the Eighties, Nineties and early Noughties, and realise this was the crest of a wave.

I wasn't at Twickenham for the aforementioned win against England, but I do remember being at the then Millennium (now Principality) Stadium for other Wales matches in that historic tournament. Sometimes I was lucky enough to go with work and host guests on behalf of ITV Wales. Sometimes I was fortunate enough to be invited by other people.

It wasn't too long after that tournament that Lee Byrne – who already seemed to be popping up in all sorts of parts of my life – started following me on Twitter and replying to a few of my tweets. I was engaged at the time to someone in England (practice makes perfect, remember?) and so, bar a small flurry of excitement (it was Lee Byrne, after all!), I thought nothing more of it.

During the next two years I split from my fiancé after it became clear things wouldn't work out longer term if we couldn't resolve how to reside in the same country. I spent a few months wallowing in self-pity at being 31 and single. Then another few months proving to myself that I could have lots of fun being single and life was good. After all, the serial monogamist in me hadn't experienced much of this! But then another few months passed, and I realised this was the time to regain some focus.

I did two things. I threw myself back into work again. And I began exercising again. I was training in the gym and preparing for a half marathon. Looking back, I do think one affected the other. As I found my stride with my running, I was finding my stride more and more at ITV. After a break-up that had left me questioning my decisions and my direction, I now had goals again, on both fronts. And it wasn't long before I found myself having conversations about presenting the national network news at the weekends.

Things stepped up a gear. Not satisfied with a half, I signed up for the New York Marathon, spurred on too by raising money for Macmillan Cancer Support after the

1. Touch. Pause. Engage.

passing of my aunt. I was definitely in the groove and moving on, forging a new life in Wales on my own.

Then one Friday evening, whilst in this groove, I was driving to London for a shift on the network news. It was a week before I was due to fly to New York. During the journey, a direct (private) message popped up on Twitter. I glanced down and saw it was from Lee. He was asking me out for a drink, 'if you're single'.

Being a sceptical journalist, I was naturally cautious about its authenticity and I thought it might be his friends messing around, so I ignored it. Later, another message came through, this time on Facebook. Also privately. He was persistent. I liked it. It wasn't long before we arranged to go for a drink once I'd returned from the marathon in New York.

A few more dates passed and it emerged that having gone from one relationship where distance was an issue, I was in danger of getting myself into another one. On our first proper dinner date, Lee announced to me that he had just signed a contract with a club in France, Clermont Auvergne, for the next three seasons. I went home not sure what to think. I think at that point I was happy to let excitement mask reality. There were friends to be introduced to, parties to celebrate and weekends being whisked away at the last minute – though only when he happened to have an injury and couldn't be selected. I also didn't fully appreciate what a contract in France meant. It wasn't like any other job where he could fly home every other weekend and I could fly there in between. There were no weekends off – in fact there was very little time off at all. I had no idea how intense a rugby season is from the inside.

31

He knew all too well, though, and he wasn't about to risk the relationship drowning in the distance of the Channel. You'll remember that I told you Lee is the antithesis of me when it comes to decisions and risks. Well, this should put that in perspective for you. Less than five months after we met, he asked me to marry him. To use an old rugby scrummaging term which the legendary newsreader (and a mentor of mine) Alastair Stewart wrote on our social media post at the time: 'Touch. Pause. Engage.'

And so within another ten months, I was walking down the aisle of a small chapel on a country estate in Mid Wales. I had filmed a story at Glanusk near Crickhowell in Powys and I'd decided there and then that, if I ever married, this was going to be the place. It was beautiful, without a doubt, but what swayed it for me was actually one practical factor: it's possible to hold your wedding in the chapel in the grounds and then it's just a short walk up a slope to a marquee on the lawn of the main house. No faffing around travelling between venues, just straight to the wedding party. For some reason, this was how I chose my wedding venue before I'd even met my husband.

'Whirlwind romance' is an overused phrase but ours undeniably was. 15 months from first date to wedding vows. And I guess it really was the stuff of fairytales. Our love story was reported in the newspapers. And with a World Cup year just past, which had seen Lee playing for his country, coinciding with me anchoring the network news frequently, our nuptials even appeared in the internationally renowned glossy lifestyle magazine *Hello*, with the headline 'Andrea Benfield makes news as she weds rugby hunk Lee Byrne'. I think we'd also hit a sweet spot in the media when people were hungry for wedding news generally, William and Kate having tied the knot the spring before.

What we couldn't have predicted was that our vows that day – for better, for worse, for richer, for poorer, in sickness and in health – would be tested to their limits over the first decade of our marriage. And as our infertility drama played out, I remember seeing the royal couple of the moment have one baby and then another baby and then another baby. I, however, remained barren.

In April 2012, we'd been together around 18 months, and married for around three of those. Lee had made it clear he wanted children sooner rather than later. If you are reading my picture of Lee correctly, you might realise that 'soon' really meant immediately! And I was pretty well in alignment with this, I suppose. We made the decision to come off the contraceptive pill, which I'd been taking for many years, and I remember thinking that I'd better bargain for getting pregnant straight away when I stopped it. I even remember pondering what that might mean for work, for marriage, for life. For where I might spend my maternity leave. Would I be giving birth here or in France?

I truly expected my body's reproductive system to start right back up again with a few turns of the ignition, despite it not having been operational in over a decade of birth control. A crude analogy, but one I've heard used by fertility experts. It hadn't crossed my mind that my reproductive engine just wouldn't know how to run any longer. But, at the start, we decided it must just be a matter of timing. Lee, as I said, had a contract in France

33

with Clermont Auvergne – notoriously difficult to get to, and even more difficult for me to get the leave granted from work to coincide with fertile windows in my monthly cycle! What's more, the stress of trying to make these dates coincide and the travelling back and forth for sex was perhaps enough to put any egg and sperm off a meeting.

After a while, we felt we needed to take some kind of action to get things moving – and that things not moving must be down to the ovulation window not coinciding with the trips I'd planned, or because I was too stressed with the mania of travelling back and forth for my body to be receptive. For those not familiar with how these things work, a woman usually releases one egg per month – just one. And it is there, ready for a little sperm to pierce it and wriggle inside it, for about 24 hours – that is all. Sperm, on the other hand, can last inside a woman for maybe five days. So all is not lost if you have intercourse in the days leading up to ovulation, but if you miss the ovulation and you are on the other side, chances are the egg has gone.

So what could we do to overcome the hurdles of distance? Well, it may sound slightly drastic, but it seemed a practical solution. We opted to go to a private fertility clinic and have Lee's sperm frozen to allow us to have what's known as an IUI: intrauterine insemination. Much like a cow is artificially inseminated with the sperm of a prize bull – or perhaps I'm bigging Lee up a little too much there! However, you know what I mean. This sounded simple. So I would use ovulation kits to determine when I was ovulating, the sperm would be defrosted, and the artificial insemination would take

1. Touch. Pause. Engage.

place. I'd stay in Wales and do it without needing to revolve flight schedules and leave from work around my menstrual cycle, and Lee would stay in France while his little tadpoles did all the work back here after warming up and waking up.

Little did we know that it wasn't quite as simple as signing up to freeze the sperm and then timing the insemination correctly. There were several appointments at a private clinic in Cardiff before we got anywhere near that point. Fortunately, Lee was somehow able to come home to do these, although I'm not sure how.

I remember our first time in the clinic's lobby area was quite surreal. This particular place was like an upmarket hotel with plush sofas, expensive artwork and shiny chandeliers. Especially in the meet-and-greet area, it was far removed from a hospital environment. Perhaps this is to justify the amount of money you are destined to hand over and to help you convince yourself you are in some kind of privileged position to be here. When really, if you are undergoing any kind of fertility treatment, it is usually completely the opposite.

The other thing that struck us was the photographs of babies all over the place. The clinic's success stories. Looking at those pictures was strange. I did feel partly that it was inappropriate to display what other people had come out the other side with, when actually the entire process is a gamble. It even provoked some feelings of envy and resentment towards those that had 'won'. However, it also brought alive the competitor in me. These other people have had babies: they've been successful. So, goddammit, why not us? My inherently stubborn personality showing up, I guess. I thought if

35

there was a possibility of it happening – of 'winning' – then I would persevere to make it happen.

But it should always be remembered that any fertility clinic is really one big casino. You have to realise that although you are a customer, you are more placing a bet than purchasing something to take home. 'Purchase', strictly speaking and according to the dictionary, means to acquire something by paying for it. So yes, you are purchasing the treatment, but you aren't purchasing the result of the treatment. When I think about the labyrinth that the clinic resembled, this gambling metaphor rings even more true. I am reminded of being in Las Vegas for my 30th birthday and I recall how they design the huge casinos so it's not easy to find the exit. Maybe this was the same. Once you've bought in, you've bought in. And even if I'm not talking about not being able to exit physically, I'm definitely talking emotionally. Betting on fertility treatment can easily become an addiction, that's for sure.

For Lee and me, at the very start of the gamble, that initial appointment was a very uncomfortable experience. We sat in the luxury waiting area, squirming. We are generally very private people and hoped we wouldn't get recognised, because I think we felt a sense of shame about being there. But actually it should have only taken those baby pictures on the walls to reassure us that this experience was so many people's 'normal' and we were far from alone. Even so, we filled in the necessary consent forms, paid the necessary fees, had the necessary blood tests – and then couldn't leave quickly enough.

At that point I was told I also needed to book in to have a procedure to check my fallopian tubes were not

1. Touch. Pause. Engage.

blocked for any reason. These are the tubes which allow the egg to travel out and away from the ovaries to be met by the sperm (hopefully). That procedure is called a hysterosalpingogram (HSG). It's a special type of fertility X-ray where iodine-based dye is placed in through the cervix by inserting a speculum (the kind usually used for a smear test), and the fallopian tubes can then be monitored for blockages and the shape of the uterus can also be assessed. The X-rays are taken by a machine lowered down over your abdomen. It's fairly painful and I'm sure anyone who has ever had any kind of fertility treatment will agree, but it seems it's a rite of passage as soon as you go down the treatment road.

No longer could Lee come to the appointments with the demands of rugby in France as they were – although I felt this was when I needed him the most, as it was the first time I'd experienced anything so invasive to my body. I'd been lucky enough never to have needed any kind of surgery. I'd broken my ankle twice, when I was 8 and (I think) 15. But, other than that, I'd barely ever needed to even visit a hospital. I suppose Lee, on the other hand, was well-versed with hospitals and surgeries. Being a rugby player, he'd already had injuries that had meant him going under the knife on several occasions. So in hindsight, from that angle, he probably wondered what all the fuss was about.

It was a strange day for another reason, too. I remember getting to the clinic in the centre of Cardiff and it was International day. Wales were playing Australia, and Lee was not in the squad for the first time. Due to WRU concerns about losing International players to clubs in Europe, he was one of those who had consequently been sidelined, having decided to play in France. Lee was caught in an unusual time regarding this problem. It was a new phenomenon that the Welsh Rugby Union was having to deal with and it turned out it would take years to be resolved. There would eventually be a new deal with the regions around central contracts, with only a select number of players who had chosen to play outside Wales being allowed in the squad, and them needing to have a certain number of caps already to qualify. But for players in 2012 it was an almost impossible time to try to navigate playing abroad *and* getting a place in the Wales squad. I remember walking through the city centre and feeling that people did not understand why I might not be excited about the game. In Wales, as I said, it's a religion. But when you see rugby from the player's perspective, you often see something very different.

Lee was dealing with all those emotions, which might seem trivial to the outsider. After all, it's just a game, right? But the pressure is so intensified inside the bubble and especially with the irrepressible noise of social media armchair critics, you become almost paranoid about everything. Whilst he was coping with that, I had my own things to worry about...

I stayed the night with my good friends Siân and Norman. They knew I had arranged to meet my mum the next day, but at this stage I didn't explain what for. In fact, she was arriving by train into Cardiff so she could be with me at the clinic.

All went well and I felt rather proud of myself for getting through an intrusive, uncomfortable and undignified examination. Little did I know that this was just the start of me losing all sense of control over my own body.

1. Touch. Pause. Engage.

The next step was the IUI that I spoke of earlier. The bit, you may remember, where I am inseminated with Lee's sperm, which has been on ice.

To prepare my body for this, I was given drugs over a period of time. The medics use the drugs to take control of your menstrual cycle, if you like. Their aim is to control when you ovulate – when you release your egg – so that they can insert the sperm at the optimal time and give the best chance of a sperm and egg meeting and fertilisation happening, so as to create an embryo. They are also aiming to control how thick your womb lining is, in order for it to be in the best possible state for that embryo to implant.

I was injecting the drugs to stimulate my follicles (where the eggs are released from) and I was taking oestrogen tablets to thicken the uterine lining. Really, at this stage I had no reason to be nervous – remember, we were only doing this to solve the issue of us not always being in the right place at the right time, and we had every confidence that the very first roll of the dice might well be lucky. At this point there wasn't a medical problem identified that we were trying to solve, just a practical one of timing.

Then there was a moment. Of all the hundreds of appointments I have had, which all blur into a mess of disappointment and hopelessness in my subconscious, this one has stuck in my consciousness because it was the very first time I had my hopes ripped from me, screwed up and tossed into the rubbish. After this, I gradually stopped bringing my hopes to any appointments or treatment cycles. This was where that protection mechanism kicked in.

It was a routine scan which ended up being everything but. I had gone in to check the progress with the follicles and the lining and find out when the IUI might be able to happen.

Instead, I was told in quite a routine manner that the IUI was not going to happen at all. The IUI was cancelled. The entire treatment cycle was cancelled. The scan showed my lining was not, for some unknown reason, responding to the oestrogen. No explanation given. There was a chart – I remember that – which had little blobs on it to chart the follicles developing on each ovary, which had been exciting. And there was another part of the chart that tracked the lining. I was told that the National Institute for Health and Care Excellence (NICE) did not recommend a transfer with a lining below 8 mm. Mine was just 4.5 mm. No more time to discuss. As I remember it, it was then thank you and goodbye.

All those drugs, all that cost, all those hopes.

All that naivety.

There were two things I remember being advised to do next. And I think I was so overwhelmed by a problem having been identified, and the fact that I was in Wales dealing with it in Lee's absence, that I just wanted to do anything I was advised to do, and quickly. What I didn't see at the time was that I was being coaxed into a fertility maze which I wouldn't escape for many years.

Firstly, I was advised to have an AMH blood test. This test is fairly well known to others frantically trying to navigate said fertility maze. It's short for Anti-Müllerian Hormone test and is meant to test your ovarian reserve. So, a measure of roughly how many eggs you have left, done through allocating a number. My number was 0.8.

1. Touch. Pause. Engage.

At that time, I had no idea what this meant. But the consultant told me over the phone that it meant that, effectively, I didn't have much time left. I remember finishing that phone call with sheer bare panic as my main emotion, which tore along quickly, gathering guilt up with it. I'd allowed myself to be late to everything in life – this was my fault: I'd failed. And then confusion rolled in too. What was meant to have been a straightforward insemination procedure to allow us to fall pregnant had led to diagnoses which would change our lives for a long time, if not forever.

And so we moved deeper into the maze. Deeper into the puzzle. And we were quickly on to the next procedure, an investigation inside my womb, which would potentially identify any issues which might be preventing the womb lining from thickening. This was called a hysteroscopy. It was treated by the medics as a very routine procedure and would take about 15 minutes under a general anaesthetic. But I didn't feel comfortable with it. During that 15 minutes, things like 'scraping' would take place. I distinctly remember that verb being used. My instinct was to recoil. If my womb lining was thin anyway, what possible good would 'scraping' it do? It felt like that was the exact opposite of what it needed. Surely it needed to be nurtured to grow, not for anything that *was* there to be scraped out for investigation? The surgeon promised that this would only be done gently or as little as possible. I can't really remember which. However, that did not provide much reassurance to my racing mind.

At this point, I felt well and truly trapped. There was no going back. We surely had to take the advice that was presented and roll with it. So I went for the operation, with my mum as my cheerleader again, as Lee was unavoidably stuck in France.

On top of the 'scraping' anxiety, which I simply couldn't remove from my mind, I was also concerned about the general anaesthetic. I must be far from the only one who has a fear of being put to sleep, and this was demonstrated when the anaesthetist came into the room and said to me, "I know what you're worried about – I'm either going to give you too much or too little." And yes, of course, that was it in a nutshell.

I had the op. I wasn't given too much or too little. I survived! The report was normal. We were still none the wiser. And this would be the first of many, many anaesthesias.

What did we know at this point? We had been told my egg reserve was low and my lining was thin. Both fairly significant developments. Both adding many a twist and turn to the maze. I went back to the clinic for a follow-up visit with one of my best friends, Carl, to try to have a discussion about where to go next. At that point, I felt my world was crumbling a little. This was no longer a case of *choosing* to pay to try to fix a practical long-distance relationship issue. This was now a medical problem. This was life giving us lemons from which it might be hard to make lemonade.

At this point, IVF was spoken about in earnest by the consultant for the first time. I knew IVF wasn't going to solve the lining issue easily, if at all. But I thought it sounded as if it would be beneficial to leave one less thing to chance. If we knew we had secured the embryos, we could work on the lining part as a separate project. That seemed practical.

1. Touch. Pause. Engage.

This navigation of the beginner's area of the fertility maze was all happening alongside quite a full-on career. Workwise, I had gone from reading the UK's breakfast news, being part of the presenter line-up for ITN's rolling coverage of the Royal wedding and the Diamond Jubilee and screen-testing for a new network morning programme to flailing around wondering what to do next. Slowly but surely, this was the beginning of fertility problems overshadowing my career ambitions. I had to make some big decisions – which I didn't realise at the time would have such an impact on my future as a broadcaster, but they really did. Because what we didn't know was how long the journey to parenthood would be, or whether we would ever arrive there. I recently saw a post quoting the former US Secretary of State Madeleine Albright, who said, "Women can have it all. Just not all at the same time." Did this hold more truth than I realised?

It was the beginning of a gradual understanding that a family was not going to come easily to us and that I would probably not be giving birth at 34, the age my mum had had me. I was dealing with the beginnings of what would eventually consume me as types of failure on two levels: my career aspirations, and my personal ambitions of starting a family. Yes, I expected to be late to the parenthood party, but I always thought I'd secure an invite, accept and off we would go. But, at this point, the party seemed off limits.

Chapter 2

The infertility vortex

IN THE FIRST year or so of not being able to conceive, there's a scatter-gun approach. And I'm not talking about ejaculation! It's what I think I'll call a Level 1 reaction on the learning curve of infertility. At this stage, you know very little. You are an impressionable blank canvas.

You want to try anything that anyone suggests which feasibly might improve things. Every vitamin and supplement available; banning caffeine; cutting alcohol; reducing stress; getting a puppy; getting two puppies; acupuncture; yoga... getting three puppies. And in parallel to all of this, you start googling for answers, for fixes, and inevitably then self-diagnosing. Yes, we all know Dr Google can feel very real.

Everyone starts on the edges, where it's safe and the sites are apparently scientific. You are just looking to try to confirm the facts about a theory you heard or a tip you were told about. Or you just want to read up a little more on what the GP or specialist might have said to you in your often all too short consultation.

But by then, of course, you've already typed whatever it is you needed confirmation on into the search engine and you've already clicked on all the clinics and private hospitals, which might tell you what you need to know in their 'Frequently Asked Questions' sections. It's funny,

2. The infertility vortex

but their answers aren't fulfilling. Because, of course, what you want to know is that if you try this random dietary plan or that expensive herbal supplement, it is proven to work. That it will work.

And so, truth be told, you are never going to find your answer, because the person you want the answers for is *you*. You are not another person on a forum with similar problems or similar symptoms. Your physiology and menstrual cycle, the number of eggs you were born with in your ovaries, your finely balanced hormonal make-up, any of which might have the most subtle but crucial effect on your fertility, are all unique.

You are looking for a mirror image of yourself and your journey hasn't ended yet. Your story hasn't been written yet. Your destiny hasn't been decided yet. Deep down you know that the random diet or maverick treatment won't necessarily work for you the way it worked for someone else. But that doesn't stop you believing. Throwing the dice. Spinning the wheel. Searching and scouring and scrolling. Sometimes for hours. Sometimes bookmarking links. Sometimes directly messaging the authors on the thread. Always wasting hours. Always getting anxious. Often browsing way past when you should be sleeping. Always adding another weight to your weary mind as it is dragged further and further down towards the seabed of depression and despair.

Even here, slipping towards the bottom, it is possible to justify your behaviour to yourself as helpful – and to justify it to others close enough to you to know what you are doing with your time. How? Because there's validation on offer. And this we can call Level 2, perhaps. Signing up for the forums. Posting on the forums.

45

Even near the outset, you can do this. You have been trying for a certain amount of time for a family. You haven't been successful. Your story has begun. You have some credentials. You have an ID in the infertility community. No, you may not fit in with all your friends who have children and are consumed with mum stuff. But you can fit in here. Here, in the online infertility vortex. It's like some twisted networking site where it's not your social or professional standing that counts, but the number of miscarriages or IVF cycles you have had.

Let me elaborate. Each person, when they post on a thread, has their 'status' below the comment. For instance, mine at one point (quite a bit further down the road) read:

> Me 37 (lining issues 3–5mm) DH 33 (no probs).
> Nov '12 Failed IUI, Jan '13 cancelled stim IUI. Jun '13 IVF – failed transfer. 9 frozen embs. Sep, Oct, Nov '13 – 3 canc FETs (oestrogen/menopur). Jan–Feb '14 Protocol w/ HCG trigger pen – 2 emb transferred – miscarried 5 wks. Apr '14 cancelled FET on same protocol – unexplained bleeding. July '15 FET ARGC 7 mm lining – BFN. Tried acupuncture/viagra suppositories too. MRI (elevated prolactin), HSG & hysteroscopy (several) – normal.

In the real world no one would understand these 'gaming credentials', but when you are in the know, they almost become a badge of honour. How far have you come? What's your history? Why should other people trust your opinions? Of course, the longer you stay on the forums and the more you interact, the more savvy you become with the shorthand and the lingo. There is a whole new language to learn. Some of the terms (which you can also

2. The infertility vortex

read in the example above) are used commonly by medics. Let's do some quick translations to get us started.

FET (frozen embryo transfer) is when the clinicians thaw out an embryo that was previously created on a brand new cycle of IVF treatment and transfer that embryo into the womb.

IUI (intrauterine insemination) is when a sperm sample that has been given and frozen is thawed and inserted into the uterus.

PGS (preimplantation genetic screening) is when embryos which may look perfectly healthy under a microscope are tested for underlying chromosomal defects before being transferred into the womb.

HCG (human chorionic gonadotropin) is the hormone you produce during pregnancy, but also will often be referred to as a 'trigger' injection, which is administered in the final stage of an IVF cycle to prompt all the follicles which have grown eggs to release them in one go, to be collected in the egg-harvesting procedure.

Using these terms will get you kudos with your fertility friends online, as you will clearly not be a newbie. But using the acronyms which have solely been developed in the forum world will step your status up another gear. Here are a few of those to get you started.

DD: Darling Daughter
DS: Darling Son
DH: Darling Husband
BF: Breastfeeding
CP: Chemical Pregnancy
BFP: Big Fat Positive
BFN: Big Fat Negative

47

And so it goes on.

My virtual investigations took me to all corners of the globe. Once, late at night, through recommendations on forums, I found a doctor in India who specialised in thin womb lining issues. I submitted my queries to him directly and waited – almost excitedly – for his answers. The answer did come and, with it, advice. Try this procedure, try these drugs. There was always something to grasp to try to regain a sense of control. Because, after all, that's what this was largely about.

Another frantic period of internet research resulted in a telephone call with another specialist in London. This led to a second HSG procedure to look at my womb a little more carefully. Did it make any difference in the end? I don't know. But it ruled things out, and it felt good to be doing something.

There were multiple examples where seeking answers virtually led me down new real-world avenues. One of those was acupuncture, so often talked about online in relation to fertility. So I found an acupuncturist specialising in women's health who was also a Chinese herbalist, and spent weeks between bulletins or before a shift dashing along to be used as a pin cushion and then be prescribed a muddy-looking potion of Chinese herbs, which I was instructed to mix with water and drink.

It was all designed to increase blood flow and therefore get more circulating to my womb to increase the thickness of my endometrium (womb lining). I stuck with acupuncture for quite some time. If nothing else, it was incredibly relaxing. The herbs I found harder to stomach and my commitment to those waned slightly sooner. I was still having regular scans to see how my

2. The infertility vortex

lining was doing and nothing at all seemed to make it budge. It was as thin as 3.5 mm at one appointment (as I mentioned, ideally it should be 8) and it was probably then that I began to look at other things to try. That's not to say acupuncture doesn't work for some people with fertility problems, but it didn't seem to work for me.

It took a lot to exhaust the list of possibilities, though, when it came to alternative medications and therapies. I even found a hypnotherapist. I'm not sure what I thought that would do. Did I really believe my thoughts were stopping me getting pregnant? Or maybe I was just losing my mind.

Not all my ideas were quite so left-field. Perhaps rather more mainstream than hypnotherapy as a complement to traditional fertility treatment was one-to-one specialised yoga sessions. I was never a 'yogi' back then – that came later. I had dabbled a fair bit, though, so when my new friend the acupuncturist and Chinese herbalist suggested the concept of one-to-one fertility yoga to me, it did seem logical. Try to get the yin and the yang balanced and my chakras flowing!

I arrived at what I remember as a fairly run-down gym down a backstreet in a part of Cardiff I had never been to before. There were a few groups of lads hanging around under corrugated iron lean-tos with their boxing gloves and towels, having just finished a sweat session. I tried not to meet their eyes, not out of any kind of fear, but out of embarrassment at what I had signed up for – though they probably had absolutely no clue what the hall was booked for next.

Inside, I'm not sure what I expected, but it was fairly dark and depressing. Small windows, low ceilings, a

49

musty, salty smell of degrading perspiration hanging in the air and thick multi-coloured mats covering the floor. But the teacher had made every effort to put me at my ease. Candles had been lit and incense was burning.

The teacher was very nice. She was younger than me and far more bohemian (which I guess wasn't difficult). She did what she was there to do. But I didn't really feel any connection. And I think with any kind of therapy or alternative therapy, that's the key. You need to have a connection to feel as if there is an empathy present which will allow you to relax and open yourself up to the possibilities on offer. More often than not, I think, if you don't believe in the person, you won't believe in the power of the solution being proposed.

What I remember with clarity is my personal space being invaded. I'm not sure what I expected, but any yoga I had encountered before involved me – in my own personal space – contorting myself into poses as best I could, with perhaps the helping hand of the instructor on the odd occasion if I had misplaced a foot or needed to get deeper into the position to feel any benefit from it. A hand would guide or softly press here and there.

But this fertility yoga was another level of tactility. I would be wrapped, quite painfully, into some kind of ball whilst her arms and/or legs were looped through mine in some way and I would be cradled and rocked. Yes, it sounds as weird to me writing it as it does to you reading it, no doubt. I'm not sure I even told Lee I was going and I certainly don't remember telling him about it afterwards. Or anyone else, for that matter.

The other strange thing that happened – aside from feeling as though I may almost tear my groin – was a

2. The infertility vortex

discussion towards the end of the cradling and rocking which was focused on chakras and colours. I'm not sure how much I was really absorbing as the entire conversation seemed rather surreal. However, the essence of it was:

a) the colour of fertility is orange
b) you can aid fertility by visualising the colour orange
c) you can aid fertility even more by wearing the colour orange
d) you can aid fertility even more by wearing orange underwear – orange knickers, in particular.

And the line I remember is:

"Maybe think about orange underwear, in particular."

So there you have it. Orange knickers. Magic pants to get me pregnant.

There is actually a very credible yogic explanation to all this (which I appreciate more now that, years on, I have sufficiently developed my own yoga practice). Chakras are the spiritual centres or energy centres that run within the human body. There are seven of them. The chakra associated with the reproductive area is called the Swadhisthana, and its colour is orange. So, it follows that orange is the colour of fertility and, therefore, it could be a good idea to start wearing orange regularly to improve my chances of conceiving.

Typically desperate not to offend and conscious that my boundaries on personal space are far more rigid than most, I tried to remain open-minded about the positions and I attempted to feign enthusiasm for the fashion advice. And sure enough – such is the nature of the neuroses of infertility – a few weeks later, feigned enthusiasm evolved into a search in my wardrobe for anything that might be orange. After all, why not? What's the harm?

It may sound utterly desperate and ridiculous to many, but this is all part of the desperation for answers. I didn't quite get as far as orange pants, but I was close. In reality, of course, the stress of trying to fit the yoga session into my busy work schedule probably negated any benefit I could potentially reap from it. But that's not how the infertile mind works. The infertility vortex is a powerful one and sucks you in with hardly any effort, and it happens very quickly.

And although it's a place which seems out of control, it was actually where I felt in control and in good company. So, further into the vortex I was sucked. Creeping shamefully around the corridors of sites filled with a lot of disinformation, and feverishly browsing the fertility forums to feed my insecurities. I would quickly lose myself in a house of mirrors, every twist and turn causing more confusion and chaos, but the search for a way out – an answer – is too great a pull.

Sometimes, it can even be an individual – another fertility patient – that pops up in a discussion who seems to offer a way out, and makes all the time and emotional energy wasted worth it. No, they may not be *you*, with your exact symptom or problem, but they seem pretty darn close to it.

One night I was browsing on one of the most popular fertility forums, desperate for someone relatable to spring up. I was searching for 'thin lining', 'thin endometrium', 'thin lining treatment', 'implantation lining'. Barely anything was being produced on the searches, which

2. The infertility vortex

was leaving me in more frustration and distress as my problem seemed to be so rare. In the process of trying to find virtual company, I was making myself feel even more isolated than I already did.

However, I then came across a thread which was a little old but seemed to relate really closely to my diagnosis. Let's call the person who posted 'Rebecca', to protect her anonymity. She described herself as having a 'treatment-resistant lining' was talking about everything she had been through with her lining issue. It sounded as if she had had a dreadful time with several treatment failures but also pregnancy losses.

So I got in touch with Rebecca. I explained our predicament at length. It always feels good to vent – I am aware this could be viewed as wallowing in my own self-pity too, but when you know you have a sympathetic and empathetic audience, which in my case then was very rare (having told almost nobody in real life), it was just too hard to resist. I'll share with you what she wrote back the initial time, because I think it gives you an extra insight into a world to which I now seemed to belong. To offer a bit of context, remember that the NHS – then, at least – would not transfer embryos or proceed with treatment whilst my lining was still struggling so much.

Rebecca:
Don't apologise! I know exactly what it's like as hardly anyone has the same problems, so when you find someone, you want to talk about it. The ones that say, "Oh yes, I had lining issues, I went in on day 7 and it was only 7.8 mm so I drank two cups of red raspberry leaf tea and when I went back two days later it was 10.4 mm"! It takes everything you have not to virtual punch or slap them, lol.

I'm not one to believe in all the pills and supplements either. I take 600 mg of vit E (OK, 536 mg because it was the closest I could find!) daily when I'm cycling. I'm not sure it helps much, if at all, but it's one pill. I've been taking 75 mg aspirin daily for most of the year because I don't think it hurts and again it's one pill. I've just bought some l'arginine and will try that – not sure how much I will take as the dose quoted for thin lining is 6 g and as I could only get 500 mg tablets cheaply, there is no way I'm taking 12 a day!

I haven't worked in some time as we have been focussing on treatment and this can only go on so long. Personally my gut feeling is that you probably do need to take a month or two off – like me, you have been shovelling all these drugs into your system and your body doesn't know if it's coming or going.

I really don't know where I stand with my lining now – on the last cycle, using the G-CSF [granulocyte colony-stimulating factor – used to increase blood supply to the womb lining], it was under 4 mm at ec [egg collection] and after they repeated the wash, I went for a scan the following week and it was just 2 mm, and it's never been that thin. My baseline after a bleed was always about the 4 mm mark so I am now very worried about even reaching 6 mm again. I have googled it to death and there are so few options for ladies in our situation.

As it stands now, my doctors have no answers, but I am working with a consultant that will let me try pretty much anything. I do the research and tell him what I want and he gives me the prescription. One I have come across and will be trying in the new year is Tamoxifen. It may be a spectacular failure but got to be worth a try – technically it's an oestrogen blocker but seems to have an oestrogenic effect on the uterus. I found a study (stupidly small group of 3!) where they had all failed to reach 6 mm on a variety

2. The infertility vortex

of regimes and all reached at least 8 mm at transfer and got pregnant. So might as well check it off the list! I will let you know if I have any luck with this.

Please keep me posted with anything you find and I will do likewise. Feel free to message me any time, though, as I know what an isolating issue this is as there are few people that understand how very frustrating it is, because no one seems to know how to help us. And the next person that casually says to me "Will you try surrogacy then?" will get a verbal bashing!

This kind of interaction was becoming my life – and continued to be for many years, whilst mostly working full-time and trying to pretend I was a 'normal' human being who was not leading a double existence.

I was looking for something I could act upon. And her suggestion of Tamoxifen was it. I recognised the name of the drug. In fact, I thought I'd probably covered news stories on it at one time or another, though I couldn't put my finger on the details. It turned out it was a drug used in the treatment of breast cancer. What Tamoxifen does is attach itself to hormone receptors – or specific proteins – in breast cancer cells and once the medication is inside the cells, it stops the cancer from accessing the hormones it needs to multiply and grow. It's actually a SERM: 'selective oestrogen receptor modulator'.

First of all, I didn't understand how something that seemed to be designed to *block* oestrogen from connecting to cancer cells could help with my thin uterine lining, which I'd always understood would have thrived if it had, or was receptive to, *more* oestrogen.

But whilst Tamoxifen acts like an anti-oestrogen in the breast cells, in other parts of the body like the uterus and the bones, it doesn't. It acts like an oestrogen. Hence the name 'selective oestrogen receptor modulator', if you follow me.

At this point, I should remind everyone that I have no medical training and nor, as far as I know, did Rebecca. But logic suggested this was worth looking into further, so I started direct messaging her (yes, you can direct message as well – there is no end to the forums' magnetic forces!).

Much like Rebecca, I had recently found a consultant that would try things if she supported the research I had found. So, after gathering more intelligence from my online source, I put the Tamoxifen idea to her and she saw no significant risks to giving it a go. For me, it was one last shot at an exit from that infertility house of mirrors, before I might be forced to engineer an exit from work in order to concentrate fully on the puzzle of the maze. Trying to keep both going was unimaginably stressful, but equally on the work front, with my career going well, the last thing I wanted to do was take time off in another country for IVF treatment.

Unfortunately – quite quickly – this particular escape was blocked off too. Tamoxifen was prescribed and I tried it. For me, it had no effect at all on the lining when my uterus was scanned. But at least I'd ruled something out. And I will always be thankful to Rebecca for reaching out to me when I needed it. I did read this on her profile bio a while later: 'Tamoxifen/Natural Cycle BFP!!!! EDD 19th January'. Which, translated, meant she had a positive pregnancy test while taking Tamoxifen on a cycle and her due date was in January. I can only hope her pregnancy all worked out for her in the end.

2. The infertility vortex

As for us, we were still trapped. My body was failing me and my research was too. I was beginning to feel broken in body and in mind. And as we tried to work out our next move, the hits kept on coming.

In parallel to alternative therapies and my individual research, there were conventional preliminary clinical tests that we had to check off before we could be accepted for IVF and fully commit ourselves to it. These included getting extra readings of my hormone levels and – little did I know – the results would lead to one of the most nerve-wracking experiences of my life.

One of the hormones in a woman's blood which is tested is called prolactin. Prolactin is a hormone made by the pituitary gland, a small gland at the base of the brain. Prolactin causes the breasts to grow and make milk during pregnancy and after birth, and levels are normally high for pregnant women and new mothers. They are not normally high for women who are not in those categories.

I was under a UK GP and consultant and having tests, but I'd also started to consult with a doctor in France. It was looking likely that if we did move up a gear to IVF, we'd have to do it in France, where we could be together, rather than the UK, due to Lee's training and playing schedule. How I would work that out with my job hadn't yet been decided.

When the results came back from my GP, both she and the consultant in France said the same thing. Prolactin was showing as consistently high. There are only a few reasons why prolactin might be high – for example, an underactive thyroid or certain medications. The other reason is a tumour of the pituitary gland. Straight away

I was told by the doctors both here and in France: never mind IVF, the first priority was to determine what was happening inside my head. Before we could think about moving on with any treatment to have a baby, I would have to be booked in for an MRI scan to check there was not a tumour, even a benign (non-cancerous) one.

I was immediately anxious. What would this mean for the longer term? Would I be on medication to shrink the tumour? Would I need to have it removed? Whilst I tried to control my catastrophising, Lee and I decided together how to go forward. I didn't want to risk not being at least in the same country as him when I had the scan, so we decided to have the MRI in France. Also, if we were hoping to have IVF in France, it would make it more straightforward if the doctors there could have more direct access to any results they might need.

The appointment was booked at a clinic on the outskirts of Clermont-Ferrand. And during a cloudy and rainy visit to central France, which perfectly matched my frame of mind, I went off on my own to try to find the place, using a tram service I had no idea how to navigate. I muddled through the ticketing service, cobbling together some A-level French and, somehow, I was on my way.

Lee couldn't miss training that particular day. It must have been the build-up to a big match. So for this one, I was alone, but at least only a short journey away from seeing him afterwards. I really wanted to cry, feeling completely overwhelmed by my foreigner status – an isolation that was intensely magnified by the day's destination and the task before me. I'd never had an MRI scan before and didn't relish the thought of being slid statue-still into a cylinder head-first whilst the machine

2. The infertility vortex

buzzed, whirred and scanned, all the while being unable to adequately communicate my needs.

Upon arrival, I was given a locker and a gown and sent into a small changing room. All my clothes and jewellery had to be removed – including my wedding ring, which I was taking off for the first time since we'd married. Even that very simple act symbolised my loneliness that day. There wasn't much time to dwell on sentimentality, though, as quite promptly I was guided to the machine and told how to lie and what would happen. Once I was in position, a dye would be injected into my bloodstream which would help the imaging to show up whether/where there were any problems.

Considering I had experienced a type of claustrophobia when I was at school, I was uncertain how I'd react to lying in the tube for so long and trying to stay as still as possible so as not to disrupt the imaging, but that part was actually not too bad. I remember doing mindful breath work to distract myself and it was all more bearable than expected.

The biggest relief, perhaps, was that not long after the whole thing had finished and I had got dressed, I was called from the waiting room to see the results. There was no waiting. There was no tumour. Thank goodness. Surely this was now the last big hurdle before we could embark on the next part of our journey?

Well, in a way it was. It was the last big hurdle to 'qualify' for IVF treatment, if you like, and that did now seem the only route left. Which also meant finally having to confront the matter at work, something I had been putting off as long as I could. I remember organising to speak to my manager. I remember the room the conversation took place in and where we were both positioned within it, but most of the words spoken are a blur. I just remember that I got upset. At that point the conversation was more around the fact that we'd need some help and I needed a confidante in my line manager as a support. I was comforted to hear that ITV would help with what they could.

At that stage I still didn't quite fully confront the prospect of needing to be in France for a longer period of time, but Lee's schedule as a professional sportsperson just didn't allow for breaks to come home for something like this. There was no such thing as sick leave or compassionate leave, really. You played unless you were at death's door, for fear of someone else playing better in your shirt and taking it for the next game, and the next. Even if you were injured, you would train full-time to rehab yourself back to full match fitness. The more I realised this and we talked about it, the more it was clear I was facing a very difficult decision.

We had to be together for the treatment, but he could not come home. And, at that stage in our careers, his earnings were higher and he could manage to support me if I didn't work and had to have treatment in France, but the same would not necessarily be true the other way around. I was in turmoil. A choice between my career and a family. A decision lots of women face – but not usually at the stage where you have no guarantees that a family could even be a reality.

I spoke to my co-presenter at work to explain that I might have to leave my job to pursue treatment with Lee in France before I got any older. I worked with Jon closely every night and felt I could confide in him. He was very

2. The infertility vortex

understanding and he came up with an idea I hadn't even considered: perhaps I could ask for a sabbatical for six months and still return to my job where I left off. Having a career to come back to would be significantly better than having to leave the job I'd worked so hard to secure over the last ten years. It would still mean breaking away from all the network presenting I was doing, which was similar to Lee's situation in that someone else would take your spot, but that seemed a risk that might be manageable. If not, I would have to accept it over time.

Stepping away from my job was wrenchingly daunting, but it was a huge relief to plan to be in the same country as we embarked on what would be some of the toughest times of our marriage. It's very strange looking back on it, because I remember that moment of temporary relief allowing a trickle of positivity. My mind raced ahead a little with, for once, an optimistic 'What if?': 'What if the IVF works and I fall pregnant, and I'll return to work only to go on maternity leave?'

Over the year in France, and even more so beyond, IVF gradually taught me that it was easier to be a stranger to this kind of optimism.

Chapter 3

Incroyable

IN THE MONTHS building up to leaving for France, I was probably experiencing one of my most desperate times. I didn't feel I was holding it together easily at work. Yes, we had this diagnosis, but it wasn't one which any clinics liked to deal with, because there didn't really seem to be any defined solution for it. It certainly didn't fall into a category on any registration forms we had to fill in and we continued to have to tick the 'unexplained infertility' box. All that was certain was that unless my womb lining thickened, treatment wouldn't progress. You'll remember, that was the clinical recommendation from the official body, NICE.

My state of mind was in crisis, so although I knew that I was pausing a career at a high point, I felt I had no other choice than to go to be with Lee. The move was further complicated because neither of us wanted people to know what we were going through at this stage, so it felt as if we were living a bit of a lie both with colleagues and with the TV audience, spinning a line about taking a sabbatical to be with Lee as we had spent little time together since we recently married.

I kept up the charade on social media over my time in France, posting an 'Insta' life which boasted cycle rides through sunflower fields, new puppies and enviable

3. Incroyable

cuisine. People from work would comment with jibes about having to continue to endure the daily newsroom grind and put up with the inclement Welsh weather, whilst I was living the life. I was probably doing myself few favours with my facade, but the thought of telling everyone the truth – and the alternative judgements that might bring – was far scarier to me.

So I carried on with my version of 'Insta versus reality' – just never posting the reality bit. Maybe mastering this skill was the next level in the infertility game. No one saw the hormonal effects that I was trying to combat with fitness. No one saw the grief which the puppies – our baby substitute – went some way to healing. The food, the scenery, the culture: all were divine, and we certainly were not ungrateful. But none were consolation enough for the pain we were going through month by month.

Once all the preparatory checks were out of the way – baseline checks of lining and hormones – it wasn't long before we were into the treatment cycle. It was a learning process as I struggled with the language, the workflow, and the medical culture. There were times when it felt there were certainly advantages to opting to do the treatment in France (not that we actually had much option), but there were other times when I felt completely confused and swamped with things to learn, because this was our first time doing a fresh IVF cycle and producing embryos and we were doing it in a foreign country.

One of the experiences I had early on did nothing to allay my anxieties. What I hadn't fully realised about France is that most things shut down completely for the whole of August and a lot of things build up to shutting down completely in July. Can you guess when we decided that I would pack up and head over to France? Yes, that's right. July. Only once I was over there and had begun the treatment cycle did we realise the full extent of the *vacances* or shutdown period, and it turned out we were unlikely to see our usual consultant – a female doctor who we had built up something of a relationship with – until after the egg-retrieval operation.

I was sent, instead, to see an older male doctor. And to this day I'm not sure whether what happened next was normal or not for France and the way things are done there. All I know is that it had certainly never happened in the UK on my IUI or stimulated cycles.

I was in the middle of a series of appointments during my cycle when, after stimulating my ovaries with hormones, they routinely checked them to see how many follicles had grown – the more follicles, the more eggs can be harvested during the operation and the more chance you have of those eggs being mature and fertilising with the sperm in the lab.

My follicles had been checked: all appeared to be on track. Then, a little randomly, the doctor checked my breasts. He totally caught me off guard – he probably explained in French that he was going to do it and why, but that was no help to me. Whether I was being touched up, I don't think I'll ever know, but that's how it felt.

However, everything when it comes to modesty is a little bit lacking in France. Or perhaps we as Brits are just a little more prudish? Nakedness does not seem to be so much of an issue to the French. This had already come into play a little bit in the fertility clinic world. In Wales, when they go to scan you and you have to lie

3. Incroyable

legs akimbo waiting for a huge dildo-like instrument to be inserted into your vagina for the next ultrasound, my experience had always been that you got a blanket or at least some blue hospital paper to put over yourself to cover your dignity – or what's left of it. In France, not so much. The doctor's consulting room could be looking straight out onto the car park with no blinds or window frosting and still you are in the chair, legs apart with no covering. They can't, but at that point in time it certainly *feels* as if the whole world can see your lady parts.

So, this boob-touching thing may have just been a part of the examination in France. And indeed I did have the experience repeated in another country by a female nurse for a slightly different reason, therefore it wasn't unfathomable that there was a point to it. But to this day no one has ever really explained why this would have happened – what he was checking for exactly and why. And it was only a few years later, probably at the start of the whole #MeToo movement, that I got to thinking that maybe this could actually have been something more than what I had reconciled it as in my mind at the time.

You see, the funny thing with all this treatment and all this desperation is that you begin to just give your body and your mind over to it. So much is happening, there is so much invasion, so much loss of dignity, that your body already doesn't feel like your own. So why would I even be surprised about another intimate examination? It came and went and I didn't even mention it to Lee.

On the other hand, there were some parts of being in France for the treatment that felt luxurious in comparison to the brief experiences I'd had in the UK. Their equivalent of the NHS would organise for a nurse to come to your house to help with your injections. The drugs being injected were to stimulate your ovaries to produce a higher-than-normal number of follicles, plus another drug to make sure you don't over-stimulate and release the eggs too soon. There's also another drug further down the line to override the one that is telling your body not to release them, because once you have stimulated enough, then it does become the time to release them! Following, so far?

During a cycle, it's common to be doing two injections a day and some are quite complicated to understand. Whereas you may have some that come pre-prepared in a syringe, which you just inject as a one-off, for most of them you are given a pack of syringes and you have to draw the right amount up each day from the vials and inject at the right time.

As I now realise, when you are an IVF veteran, this all becomes part of the everyday. But what is second nature to me now was incredibly confusing back then, as a complete beginner who was also trying to understand it all in a different language, with a dyslexic husband. So the mobile nurse was a very welcome sight on the doorstep.

Aside from the dubious breast examination incident, everything went smoothly in the initial stages of that first round of IVF, for which we were very grateful. Once the stimulation injections were complete, then came what I was talking about before – an injection to tell the follicles to release the eggs, otherwise known as the trigger injection. From there, within a very specific number of hours I had to be at the hospital for a general anaesthetic to collect the eggs from the follicles.

3. Incroyable

I was separated from Lee for the procedure itself, as you would expect, as I was taken to an operating theatre. I felt particularly vulnerable removing my glasses on this occasion (usually I would wear contact lenses – but that, of course, wasn't allowed for surgery). My eyesight is terrible without my specs and I can barely make people out. My ability to communicate already felt depleted because I didn't speak the language well, so to have another of my senses severely reduced was daunting. However, within a few minutes I would be deeply asleep, so I just hoped my glasses would be there by my side when I woke up.

When I did come round, it wasn't long before I was told how many eggs had been collected. It seemed to be OK, although at this stage I had nothing to compare it to. 18 were collected, 14 of which were considered to be mature – in other words, they had grown and developed as much as they needed to to have a good chance of fertilisation in the lab. Now we would wait for a few days to see how many of the eggs would fertilise.

Which brings me to the part that I actually know very little about, but which it's very important not to ignore. The eggs would be fertilised in a petri dish in the lab with Lee's sperm, which had already been collected. This is actually the only physical part that the man has to get involved with if the woman is the one with the fertility issues. The deed is done in a private room with appropriate material to hand. I think that's all I want to say! Suffice to say, we've never really talked about it in any great detail.

There was an added layer of clinical intervention with my eggs and Lee's sperm. They wouldn't just be left to see if they fertilised on their own – which is the way with traditional IVF (in vitro fertilisation) – in our case ICSI (intracytoplasmic sperm injection) would be performed. This means that the sperm is injected directly into the egg, to give a better chance of successful fertilisation. It's a laboratory process for which you need a very steady hand! And one which Lee was even invited to go to observe. I remember the doctor in charge of the embryology side of things in our case was a rugby fan (as were 99% of the population in Clermont-Ferrand), and he asked Lee if he wanted to have a show and tell in the lab. Lee is much more of a visual learner, so I think it was really great for him to be able to understand the process better, and have a little more empathy for my experiences too.

Behind-the-scenes tour complete, just two days later we had decisions to make. Out of the 14 mature eggs, 9 had fertilised to form embryos, which seemed like a good result. However, the embryology team was reluctant to allow us to have an embryo transferred back into my womb, because – guess what? – my lining was not thick enough. And so it began in France as well. They would cancel the treatment because the endometrium was too thin. What on earth were we here for, if they were never going to be able to transfer the embryos back? It was like having what seemed like all the perfect ingredients for a cake, but the oven never being ready to cook it.

We begged them to reconsider due to the problem with my lining being long-standing, and explained that the 6.5 mm it had reached on this cycle was, for us, fantastically good. It was a long time waiting for that call, but in the end they said they would transfer one embryo

3. Incroyable

to my womb and freeze the other eight. We breathed a big joint sigh of relief. Significant progress. Something to note here – in France at the time they worked on a different premise to most of the UK. They froze our embryos on Day 2 after they were fertilised. The norm in the UK is to let them develop in the lab until Day 5, to see if they become what's called a blastocyst. This is when an embryo is slightly more advanced. The belief is that it has better chances of implantation and pregnancy if it is transferred as a blastocyst. However, there are other schools of thought, which I guess France adhered to at the time, which assumed that an embryo is best put back as soon as possible into the womb, where it would be in the case of a natural pregnancy. Again, take my medical commentary with a slight pinch of salt. But I gather that is the general difference in thinking, and research has been done in both methods.

It's extraordinary, over time, what your memory decides to retain. There are many moments that are still vivid recollections with regards to test results or turning points in treatment but I don't have any memory at all of where we were or what I felt when we had the first result from this first round of IVF. We must have taken a test but I don't know if that was a blood test at the hospital (the usual routine in a treatment cycle in France) or a normal 'pee on a stick' pregnancy test at home. Maybe we didn't really expect it to work the first time and so the disappointment, though it must have been there to a degree, hasn't particularly stuck in my mind, like so many other disappointments have.

What does stick in my mind is the wider impact of our inability to conceive. In many ways, it was far more

69

stinging in France because of the environment I was living in there. Many of the players were international – from New Zealand, Australia and South Africa, for example. We found ourselves gravitating, rightly or wrongly, to these players and their families as our social group, because we all spoke English and because we all had the shared experience of being away from home, I suppose.

What I also found in this group was that, because the women had all made a decision to come with their husbands whilst they played out their contracts, this was the perfect time for them to have babies. After all, they'd had to move away from home and career prospects to be on the other side of the world, so the obvious next move was to fulfil the ambition of becoming a mum instead. So, bar one other player's girlfriend, who was also from the UK, every woman was either pregnant or had one or multiple very young children.

On match day, as a wife or partner, you could have access to a family room to watch the match. But I could think of nothing worse than being stuck in a glass box full of babies and young children. I've nothing against other people's children, but for me then it was mental torture. A weekly reminder of what I considered to be my failure and a breeding ground for questions about my lack of offspring. Quite often I'd decide to use the ticket we also had for the outdoor stands. And as anyone knows who has ever spectated for a rugby season, it was inevitably freezing, or freezing and wet. It would also have been in danger of being very lonely had it not been for Rachel, the then girlfriend of one of the French players that I mentioned, who would also often choose to be outside.

3. Incroyable

We shivered along together and have remained firm friends ever since. And actually, despite the inclement conditions, it was always a better atmosphere to hear the cheering crowds and the beating drums, instead of being inside with the ambience tempered by glass.

I don't say all this to sound bitter and twisted. I say it more to emphasise the isolation that comes with infertility. An isolation which anyone who has had it touch their lives will immediately recognise. An inability to go to baby showers; turning the other way rather than bump into the pregnant colleague at work (sorry to you – I think you know who you are!); quick exits when someone arrived in the office with their new baby – none of these things came from a place of nasty jealousy but instead from a place of utter devastation at my own failings, a crippling fear that I may never be a parent because of them and a deep guilt that I would also deny that privilege to Lee.

Whilst the intensity of the rugby family in France had its curve balls for us, it did also prove an invaluable network. As you may already have gathered, Clermont-Ferrand was on another level when it came to supporting its rugby club. Every game was like going to an International. It was incredibly exciting to be in the Stade Marcel-Michelin on match day. And with that fierce loyalty to the sport in the city came a fierce loyalty to the players. Support was everywhere and when those in the medical community who were fans got wind of our struggles, they wanted to help, make suggestions, give recommendations. It had felt up until this point, both in the UK and in France, that no one really knew how to treat my thin lining so when, as a result of some of those conversations, it was suggested that we talk to another consultant who might have some ideas, we decided that was a good move.

We started going to a different hospital in a different part of town, to a man who was deemed to have a great deal of experience in complex fertility issues. And he did come up with some experimental ways to try to thicken the lining. First of all I took a different type of oestrogen called synthetic oestrogen, which he thought my body might react to positively, as it had no reaction at all to the typically prescribed oestrogen. We tried it, but the cycle ended up again being cancelled, because the lining did not thicken to an acceptable level for implantation to be successful. A pattern was emerging, and not one I wanted to continue.

I was holding on to the positives though. It *was* good that the new doc was trying new things which were outside the box. And each time we visited his clinic, I sensed he'd contemplated further since our last appointment, and developed a new plan. It was fortunate that his medical knowledge was so respected, because I couldn't say quite the same for his bedside manner. We would arrive and he would greet Lee enthusiastically with handshakes and *bisous* – kisses on both cheeks. Once again, he was a big Clermont Auvergne rugby fan. I was not a rugby player.

He greeted me also, though not so enthusiastically. I knew my place, and that was to go to the big chair, strip off the bottom half of my clothing and lie back, feet in the stirrups, whilst he chatted to Lee about the last game and the next game, the last season and the next season, the last coach and the new coach. A conversation that

3. Incroyable

was held partly in his broken English and partly in Lee's broken French. I'm sure he learnt very little about team tactics, but I'm not sure he cared. He had a story to tell his friends.

All the while, I am waiting there, legs akimbo. Eventually, the chatter comes to a close and my existence is again acknowledged. Though barely. More just my lower half, really, as he prepares the vaginal probe for the ultrasound and inserts it. Attention is then turned to the monitor, which shows the intra-vaginal ultrasound scan in the usual grainy black and white. It's hard to make anything out but by this stage I know what I'm looking for. My eyes go straight for the lining and I try to gauge its thickness.

It's thin. But I wait for official recognition of this. Each visit it's the same. I know precisely what's coming.

"*Incroyable.*"

And again. "*Incroyable!*"

"*C'est quatre millimètres seulement. Incroyable. Incroyable.*"

"Unbelievable. Unbelievable. It's only 4 millimetres. Unbelievable!"

Not even this exclamation of disbelief at the rarity of the specimen he saw before him did he direct at the person directly involved. I may as well have been under general anaesthetic for all the attention he was paying to me as his patient.

I'm sure this was not done maliciously and quite possibly was borne out of a social awkwardness or shyness to communicate. I've no idea, but what I didn't quite need in those moments was to be treated like a fascinating but freakish experiment.

However, for all his communication shortcomings, Mr *Incroyable* did come good again with a fresh idea. You may remember me talking about the 'trigger injection' of the hormone HCG (human chorionic gonadotropin), which releases the eggs from the follicles of the ovaries when they seem ready to be collected during an IVF cycle. Well, Mr *Incroyable* had a theory that using a very tiny bit of this hormone every day during part of my cycle might be worth a try, to see how the lining responded. Yep, why not? Seemed to be worth a go if we were ever to get to the stage of having an embryo transferred. So this is what we did next.

I was once again pumped with hormones – the HCG shot now being an added ingredient in the recipe. Then the embryos were thawed on the appropriate day. One didn't survive the initial defrost – which sometimes happens – so we thawed another. The lining had increased minimally, the transfer was done and we waited.

If you are familiar with trying to conceive on any level, you will be familiar with the 'two-week wait'. This is the two weeks from when you ovulated and had sex, if you are trying to conceive naturally – or, if you're having IVF, from the time you transferred an embryo/embryos. It's an agonising fortnight during which your body tries its best to trick your mind that you are pregnant and vice versa. Then the next day, you are convinced you are not, because the symptom or the optimism or both have diminished. Nothing you do to try to distract yourself works and everything you do, you question. Should you be having that glass of wine? Should you be having that cup of tea? Would that argument you had last night affect the result?

3. Incroyable

The test we did on this occasion was a blood test, and we picked the results up via a patient portal online. This was better than having to ring, considering the considerable language barrier. We kept checking for updates until eventually a result had been uploaded. Now, if there's an HCG level in your blood above 5 mIU/mL, then that could be a pregnancy. Our result was 8.

It was then that we learnt that there is a wait more agonising than the two-week wait. Our consultant Mr *Incroyable* said, "Something has happened." But he wasn't sure what. Even in the very early days of pregnancy, the HCG level should be a lot higher than 8, so we would have to sit it out with blood tests every two days to see if the pregnancy was 'viable' – an absolutely terrible word. In essence, whether the embryo would develop and survive any longer.

The HCG levels were meant to double every two days. And they did continue to creep up until they got to just above 30, as far as I can remember. But when we compared this to the tables online, I think both Lee and I knew this was not where things needed to be. And eventually the numbers diminished again. It's what's termed a chemical pregnancy – technically, a very, very early pregnancy loss. I started bleeding shortly afterwards.

Just for that week or so when we thought we had achieved a conception – after two and half years of trying – tension departed for just a little while. There was a huge sense of relief.

Mr *Incroyable* said he couldn't be certain if the HCG reading had been from a residue of the hormone which we had been drip-feeding from the trigger injection. If so, that might have caused a false result. But even he said it was unlikely it would have continued to build before tailing off completely.

It seemed we had had a pregnancy, of some kind. So what now?

In the background, my quest to find answers through the internet continued. Whilst all the action had been going on in the foreground with experimental treatment cycles, cancelled cycles, failed cycles, I had been continuing to seek advice from internationally renowned scientists who specialised in thin endometria. One of those was based in California and I'd organised for us to have an initial video call with him to see if he might be able to help.

One thing he was adamant about was that unless we could get my lining to 8 mm (remember, at points it had barely been 4 mm), then he didn't believe a pregnancy would implant sufficiently to be 'viable' (again, yuck).

But he did suggest two things. Firstly, he wanted me to send my blood to a special lab in the USA where they would test for 'natural killer cells'.

The more we ventured down this infertility road, the more we heard about these NK cells. It seemed to be a thing. Essentially, if you had a high level of NK cells in your blood, then there was a higher chance that your own immune system would reject the embryo as a foreign body trying to attack. That's a very crude description, but I think accurate.

We ordered a pack from America. I somehow organised to go to a private clinic where I could pay for them to take my blood and then I had to send the sample back within a strict amount of time to a lab in Chicago.

Tick.

3. Incroyable

Secondly, he suggested a novel treatment, but one that seemed to be logical. And one that his clinic, he said, had had success with in terms of increasing the lining.

Viagra.

Yes, you heard me right. Viagra.

How, I hear you ask, does that work? Viagra, I hear you say, is for male impotence. Well, it is, yes. But how does Viagra work? It works by increasing blood flow to the necessary male organ and creating an erection. Mr California's theory was that it would work on that same premise in a woman and increase blood flow to the womb, and therefore the lining.

His clinics had even created a Viagra suppository so that women could insert them directly into the vagina and it would be absorbed into the blood in the right area of the body, rather than having to be taken by mouth. Makes sense. Well, I thought it did.

Viagra suppositories ordered from America. At a huge cost. Obviously.

Tick.

Thanks Mr California.

It turned out getting Viagra suppositories into France from America was not as easy as I'd hoped it might have been. Perhaps it was because we were binge-watching *Breaking Bad* at the time, but the rigour of the customs process made me feel very much like an illegal drug smuggler. And then there was the added layer of complication of trying to explain to French customs what it was, what it was actually for and why I was having it sent to me from the States. Eventually it arrived.

We used the suppositories on the next cycle with more oestrogen – pills and patches. Another gamble. Another maverick treatment. And, yes, you've guessed it, another disappointment. The lining did not thicken. 'No go' on the transfer.

I wrote back in desperation to Mr California. I explained that now we had clocked up a failed insemination and a cancelled stimulated insemination cycle due to thin lining, plus one failed fresh transfer on an IVF cycle and now a cancelled FET (frozen embryo transfer) with Viagra suppositories, oestrogen pills and oestrogen patches. I explained that I seemed to have zero response to the oestrogen and Viagra.

He did suggest one other drug combo, which we went on to try (with no luck). But it was his closing paragraph that left me speechless.

> If all fails, then the only remaining alternative will be IVF using a gestational carrier, in which case I recommend that we talk again and possibly plan on your coming to the United States for that process. It would involve your being here for no more than about 8–10 days. We could help you find a gestational carrier and help prepare her for an appropriate embryo transfer procedure down the line.

Mr California was saying he had no more answers except to help us find another woman to carry our baby. A surrogate. How had it come to this? Even world-renowned experts had nothing left to suggest.

It was the first, but not the last, we would hear of surrogacy. But at this point, I had to focus fast on what decisions to make then and there. I'd already been nearly six months away from work – which had been the original sabbatical agreement. With things as they were, and so much having gone wrong, we were still in a position

3. Incroyable

where we had embryos in storage but no answer as to how to get my womb in a position to grow them.

I started to despair. We were approaching Christmas again – a time of year I had always loved but now dreaded. An annual reminder that we had no family of our own to share in the magic. I would also need to start negotiating with work to take some more time off, if we were to try to find a way forward with the frozen embryos.

Other than the comfort of being with Lee and the endlessly present listening ear of my mum on the phone, two things saved me in those moments where it felt like all hope was evaporating. And their names were Hank and Marcy. Or Iggy and Ivy. In France, if you get a puppy, you have to register the animal with a name that starts with the letter that's being used for new births that year. They were two miniature schnauzers. Unable to succeed in bringing a baby into the world, we fell straight into the stereotype of 'infertile couple gets a dog'. Or, in our case, two. But there is a very good reason why animals are used for therapeutic purposes. Of course, they filled a void, but it was also those two little balls of fur that Lee would bring to me when I was face down, sobbing into the pillow, not knowing what to do next.

With my therapy dogs firmly established in post, what I actually decided to do next was secure another six months off work. Then, in the time we had left together in France, we did more cycles of treatment with the frozen embryos, during which we decided to transfer embryos back regardless of the thickness of the lining. At this point it felt like we had nothing to lose.

But it was more of the same – negative results and disappointments. And we returned to the UK in the summer of 2014 with no baby, two puppies and repeating the same line we had always stuck to for those that had asked about my leave of absence: we'd just wanted to be together as a newly married couple. For that white lie, I remember being trolled online. Maybe I should have seen that coming. I understand it may have looked as if I was in quite the privileged position: those with partners in the military said I should count myself lucky, and others even called me a gold digger. They weren't to know the truth of my year off-screen, of course. But still it hurt. I think if you can't say anything positive, why say anything? No one ever knows what people are going through in private, after all.

CHAPTER 4

Rugby full-time, IVF half-time

IN JUNE 2014, we were back at our home in Wales. Hank and Marcy travelled back in our car with Lee and me via the Eurotunnel. Our belongings followed in a large removal lorry, turning up a few days later.

It certainly felt like the end of a period of play as far as the fertility treatment was concerned. Half-time, maybe. A time to reassess, have some serious team talks and create a way forward. A way which might create a win for us. But what tactics could there be that we hadn't already tried? Well, after how things had been left in France, neither of us knew. I think we were a bit lost.

Lee was changing jobs. He was joining Newport Gwent Dragons and had been asked to captain the side. An exciting prospect to move on his career, but a stark change from the packed stadiums and high-profile league of the Top 14.

I was returning to relaunch a news service. We had moved to new premises whilst I'd been in France, and with that we had a new studio and a new programme. From June 2014, there would be just one presenter in the studio fronting the programme. Jonathan Hill – my co-presenter, who had been the one to suggest a sabbatical when I'd been on the verge of leaving my job – and I would take turns anchoring what would now be called *Wales at Six*.

There were new starts on all fronts. But we were still no clearer what new start there could be as far as trying to conceive was concerned.

There were different options. We had six embryos still in the freezer in France. So one of the first things I did was arrange for them to be couriered over to the UK and stored at a clinic we had looked into in London. Science and technology always impress me – that I can call up a company and they can send someone with the right kit to a clinic in France and successfully transport what were potentially our future children back home. Our most precious possessions, I suppose, at that point. They arrived safe and sound to bed in in their new freezer. We had no idea at that stage when or if they would be used, but it felt good having them there. Knowing there were possibilities. The game was not over.

We did both allow ourselves some time. I think that was non-negotiable. We needed to get back into our stride and settle back in. All the while in the background, though, I was doing research. Ever since Mr California had suggested that ultimately surrogacy might be our only option, I had been looking into what that might entail. It was complex and extraordinary, and not helped by legislation in the UK, which might have been preventing surrogates coming forward.

For a start, commercial surrogacy – paying another woman to accept your embryo into her womb and carry it hopefully through a pregnancy and a birth – is legally very tricky to navigate in the UK. It's common for arrangements to be largely altruistic and the surrogate given expenses – for maternity clothes, for instance, or trips to the hospital, and to cover loss of earnings. So

4. Rugby full-time, IVF half-time

unless you know someone such as a relative or very good friend who will do this life-changing sacrificial thing for you, you would have to find a surrogate through an organisation, because advertising for a surrogate is also not allowed. However, though they have to be non-profit, these agencies still cost money – for one. And secondly, agencies simply did not have enough surrogates coming forward. One thing that seemed to deter people was that if you carry a baby for someone, you are the legal parent and it can take months for the intended parents' parental order application to be processed and for the baby to officially be signed over to them. Any surrogacy agreements you've drawn up between you are also not legally enforceable. This issue, amongst others, meant there was little chance of 'intended parents' like myself and Lee finding a surrogate anytime soon in the UK.

Whilst I was discovering that the odds of finding a surrogate were so terrible here, Lee was starting to struggle at the Dragons with injury. In one of his home games he had suffered a dislocated shoulder and was taking a long time to come back from it. He was in pain and on a lot of drugs. I knew he wanted to play on, and he tried to, but in the end they decided to operate.

The operation went well, but when they had seen what was going on inside his shoulder, they realised the extent of the damage. To some degree he was fixed, but it did seem as if, from that point, the writing was on the wall. In the spring of 2015 he was forced to take the decision to hang up his boots. Not in the way he would have wished, with a final hurrah playing on home soil, but instead having to succumb in the battle with rehab from injury. Speak to any professional sportsperson, and none wants

83

their career to end in this way. Yet, sadly, for so many it does. For Lee and his impassioned relationship with the sport he loved, it was over. How can you prepare for the end of an era and the breaking of a thread which has run through two decades of your life? Well, not easily, especially when the game forces you to live it entirely, in order to get that winning edge. There is no time, no chance, to be thinking of the next step, the next career. There is only the next game, the next tournament.

So began perhaps the hardest year of our marriage, with Lee grieving for his career and both of us mourning the losses so far on our fertility journey. Little did we know there was further loss to come. And half-time on our fertility journey would need more than just a rousing team talk. It would need a love that would help us pull each other up from the depths of despair and a will to carry on that surpassed the ordinary. That ambition, tenacity and perseverance that had held so much attraction for me in Lee when we first met – and vice versa – would be tested more than we could have imagined.

Because on 5 June 2015 we woke up to a text from a family member with a link to a newspaper headline which read that All Black Jerry Collins had died in a car crash in France.

Jerry Collins was a rugby legend in his own lifetime, not only in New Zealand but around the world. I think that's the only way to describe him. He was unique in playing style and ability, but perhaps even more so in character. I've never met anyone who compared to him. And he was one of Lee's dearest friends.

Jerry lived with Lee in Bridgend in Wales for much of the time they were both at the Ospreys – a club Lee

4. Rugby full-time, IVF half-time

played for from 2006 to 2011, with Jerry alongside him for the last two seasons. They formed a strong bond and in the months preceding his death, Lee had been to visit Jerry in France, where he was playing for Narbonne. I know they shared conversations about Lee's retirement and he was probably one of the very few people Lee would emotionally confide in.

When we married in 2012, Jerry was his usual elusive self. He rarely stayed on one mobile number for long and it was often impossible to track him down. Nevertheless, Lee invited him anyway and hoped for the best. It was anybody's guess whether he would turn up, especially as he was playing in Japan at the time.

But a day before, Lee received word that he was travelling over and would be there. Jerry proceeded to put the incomparable Collins stamp on the event. There are a few things I remember vividly. He arrived in time to join us for a meal the evening before the wedding. I sat next to him at dinner and when there was talk of the bill and the inevitable calculations of who was paying what, he was writing the sums on his jeans. Yes, I do mean his jeans. He was working out the bill and what everyone should pay (or so I thought) on the leg of his trousers.

Then, the next thing I knew, the bill had been settled. But not by any of the immediate wedding party. Jerry had rocked up to the bar and paid for the entire thing.

I found out later that this generous act might well have been currying favour with me ahead of time. It turned out that he was – post meal – responsible for employing the services of several taxi drivers, who he asked to follow the bachelor party from drinking venue to drinking venue, where he seemed to be the ringleader

85

in getting everyone far merrier than they might have been planning – considering there was a significant event the following morning. In the morning, the groom's two best men showed up at the marquee looking sheepish, but they were adamant Lee was up and at it in the gym. They fooled me enough that when Lee greeted me at the altar looking red-eyed and emotional, I thought he was overwhelmed by the whole event and seeing me walk down the aisle. Turns out he was just incredibly hung-over. Well, RIP Jerry. All these years on, all is forgiven (just).

The car crash in France which took his life did not only involve him. His partner Alana also died, and their three-month-old baby, Ayla, was seriously injured. Reportedly, Jerry was found shielding her in the back seat to try to protect her from the impact. And protect her he did. She now lives with Alana's sister in Canada and, though she still bears the impact of the crash in many ways, she is a thriving 9 year old.

As news spread about his death – which we reported on ITV Wales – more stories emerged of Jerry's kind heart and remarkable character. One unexpected message I received came from Tiggy Legge-Bourke, former nanny to Prince William and Prince Harry, and it was another recollection from our wedding. The Glanusk Estate where we got married is owned by the Legge-Bourke family and Tiggy lives in the grounds. One of the choices of accommodation at that time was staying at the bed and breakfast at Tiggy's.

We'd reserved this for Jerry – just in case he turned up. He managed to find Tiggy's prior to the aforementioned dinner, with no one really knowing he'd arrived. And in her correspondence to me, Tiggy described how he made

4. Rugby full-time, IVF half-time

his first impression. She recounted walking into her kitchen to find a largely naked All Black standing there, having just showered after a long journey, protecting his modesty with a small towel. What he did next, though, was Jerry through and through. He managed to get himself into some clothes, and then spent time outside running through rugby drills with her children. As she said, most certainly one for the memory box.

For all whose paths had crossed with Jerry, his death was a moment when you realise the world has lost someone unique. This became more apparent as more stories emerged of his eccentric kindness and huge personality. For Lee, already feeling bereft for his career, it was a knock he reeled hard from and it would be a while before its impact would allow him to get back up and carry on.

Alongside this, we were having to make decisions about treatment as time was ticking on. I was more than aware that I was nearing my 37th birthday. According to the stats, my chances of conceiving had already fallen sharply. But, despite the issues, we did still have the embryos. Embryos made from eggs from a younger me. So there was hope. We still needed that game plan for the second half. A decision on when and how to use those embryos, and a knowledgeable doctor to help with the womb issues.

The French embryos were waiting for us in London. So this seemed the obvious next step. The clinic there was pricey, but had good stats on success and we had long given up trying to put a price on the joy of having a baby. Of creating and growing a life. Of having a legacy. So even though you know you can't actually afford it, somehow you think you can find a way. Or, in reality, you find a debt plan. You remember how I said infertility affects every part of life. Well, here's the financial hit. Yes, we'd both had good jobs, for which I was very grateful. So, yes, it was an option for us, which I am very aware it isn't for many others. But just to make it clear, unless you are earning football star or network primetime TV wages or you win the lottery, *no one* can really afford to pay for fertility treatment. It's off-the-scale money and it's not something you will have planned for in the average household budget. You know you'll be paying it back for a long time to come.

I don't say this for sympathy, because I know we were fortunate to be able to even contemplate these costs. I just say it to put in context all the comments I hear when there is a news story about a couple shelling out a shedload of money for countless cycles of IVF. Often I will hear, "Well, lucky for them – they could afford it." Well, it will always be 'afforded' with a multitude of other desperate sacrifices, in order to try to succeed in what others seem to do so naturally. And there will always be loans and credit cards involved.

The London clinic had a good reputation and its stats were amongst the best in terms of successful pregnancies. We knew it would be our last shot in terms of thinking about paying any big chunk for treatment, so we decided to go for it. The first thing they suggested was that we used one of the frozen embryos from France on another FET cycle. This can be done on many different drug protocols. It can be natural, without any drugs except basic hormones to support the cycle, and the timing of the transfer of the embryo back into my womb would be

4. Rugby full-time, IVF half-time

decided based on peeing on an over-the-counter ovulation stick to gauge the best window for implantation. Or it could be done using drugs to shut off my usual cycle and the clinic effectively taking control of it with more drugs. The latter was what we went for. They took into account my lining problem and so also chucked Viagra into the pot of medication. This time it wasn't taken as a vaginal suppository, but orally.

I think the thing I hadn't quite realised until we got closer to the treatment was just how many patients the clinic had and how – in order to process the numbers – they needed to be almost military in their procedures rather than personal and compassionate. Mr *Incroyable*, come back, all is forgiven.

First of all, prior to the start of the cycle, I was asked to attend a tutorial seminar with a group of women, to teach me how to mix up different vials of drugs which would need to be drawn up and injected at specific times of the day. It was completely surreal. All these women, gathering at the start of what was basically a fertility treatment bootcamp: getting our instructions, scribbling everything down frantically. We were being taught, in the space of about an hour, to be our own nurses. It was quite overwhelming and I realised how spoilt I'd been in France, with the help they offered there. I also found it quite sad that though we all had a common purpose, there was still very little sense of camaraderie. In our own ways, we all felt ashamed and/or resentful about being there. I did make some friendships along the way, but they were tricky as you couldn't be sure how you'd feel if they were successful and you weren't, or vice versa. The emotions were forever complicated.

The clinic did some new things too. Something called a karyotype test, which makes sure that chromosomes are not something that could be causing a problem by checking the chromosome set of both partners to rule out underlying genetic abnormalities.

The bootcamp vibe continued right up to when we approached the transfer itself. I remember getting a phone call in the ITV dressing room one evening, shortly before air, instructing me to come into the clinic the following morning at 6 a.m. as I was listed for a hysteroscopy. Little did I know, but at this clinic, having a hysteroscopy prior to your transfer was routine. It was the same op under general anaesthetic which I'd been advised to have right in the beginning, when they wanted to check if there was something more going on to cause my thin womb lining. I totally panicked: a combination of the surprise and shock at being asked to go in for a general anaesthetic with less than 12 hours' notice, my general anxiety around anaesthetic, my worries about someone scraping my uterus and the fact that I was on the roster to do the late news. If I had to be in central London for 6 a.m., and I finished work past 11, I may as well not go to bed!

Fortunately by this point I had confided in my boss' PA, the wonderful Sue, who also did the rosters and was a mastermind in finding solutions to problems. I popped my head out of the dressing room door, which opened pretty much directly onto the busy newsroom, and asked if she could come in for a few minutes. Through tears, I explained what was happening. She went immediately into solution mode. I was very lucky to have such support and lucky to be able to have it signed off at the last minute

4. Rugby full-time, IVF half-time

as well. I know there is a lot of talk at the moment about workplaces needing policies to support women's health, whether that's fertility, menopause or miscarriage. In the absence of a fertility policy, I couldn't fault the reaction I had in the moments where it was make or break in terms of whether a cycle could continue or not. There was an understanding that I *had* to put this first. It actually was life or death stuff. Maybe they also understood that these were our last chances.

I managed to get in for the op. The cycle proceeded. It felt as if every day was like this. I dripped with anxiety. Each injection was done tentatively, waiting for something to go wrong. Terrified that I'd inject the wrong amount at the wrong time, or in the wrong way. They wanted to monitor my bloods too, to check the hormone levels were as they wanted. This was done more with this clinic than any other I'd known – even for a frozen embryo transfer, they wanted a lot of checks. All we could do was assume this was a good thing. The more data, the more accurate the calls could be on when or whether to transfer.

The data apparently showed I could benefit from an infusion too. This was new. The clinic did two types of blood infusions: one costing hundreds of pounds and another, which was far more complex and cost thousands, which fortunately was not prescribed to me. I was offered the former – an intralipid infusion based on a blend of soya oil, egg yolk and glycerine, which is thought to protect the cell membranes from natural killer cells' attacks. As I mentioned earlier, there was a theory in many clinics that the womb can build up natural killer cells, which effectively meant your own immune system would kill off an embryo. I was told my bloods showed mine were borderline, so I should have the infusion. It turns out these blood tests may not tell the whole story – but more on that later. With the knowledge I had at the time, I dragged myself to the clinic and sat in its Marylebone basement, hooked up to a bag of liquid which made a huge dent in my credit card but, I was told, could be part of the success story of this cycle.

Somehow we got to the transfer stage without breaking. At one stage I remember being in Manchester for something for work and realising that I'd forgotten to get the Viagra prescription. I didn't think I'd need it the particular days I was away, but it meant Lee ended up driving around out-of-hours chemists trying to find it. Recalling memories like that, I realise what a star he was a lot of the time, and that I didn't acknowledge it enough. It can't have been easy for a recognisable British Lion to be going into pharmacies in the middle of the night begging for in-stock Viagra. But he just did it. He knew what it meant.

That year, I actually don't know how we carried on. Lee had always considered the number 15 lucky, but 2015 was our *annus horribilis*. There was the backdrop of Jerry's death and Lee travelling to New Zealand for his funeral. During those same few months, we were also coping with a close family member being diagnosed with cancer, as well as Lee trying to establish what a new career and a new identity might look like. It turned out being medically retired was no walk in the park.

We did the pregnancy test on 3 August. BFN. Big Fat Negative. Again. All that effort, all that juggling, all that emotion, all that money. How do you keep getting back up? It wasn't so easy this time.

4. Rugby full-time, IVF half-time

The Rugby World Cup was about to kick off. Somehow I hadn't foreseen that this would be a huge trigger for Lee. Combined with everything else, a World Cup being hosted in England – so exciting for so many – for us turned out to be very damaging and a massive turning point. I don't think I need to go into details, out of respect for my husband and our privacy, but as Lee mentioned in his own autobiography, he went off the rails a bit, partying as if there was no tomorrow. He just wanted to get lost in something else and on top of everything we'd been going through, London, the World Cup, encouragement from so-called friends old and new – well, it was the perfect storm. Let's just say, it almost broke us.

My work carried on as normal – hosting awards ceremonies, filming current affairs documentaries, fronting the news, trying to get new projects off the ground in London, presenting the network bulletins. In parallel, I started seeing a psychologist. I would go on my break on the late shifts or at lunchtime as it was really close to work. Often, after having been streaming with tears, I'd take a breath, walk five minutes back across the road and go on to do the evening or late news. At that point, it was treading water. It was surviving. Eventually Lee came with me. I was convinced he wouldn't show up, but he did. I'm a real believer in talking therapy and I do think it changed the path we were travelling on. We went away for a few days to Budapest in January 2016 (we had tried to go away each year around our anniversary) and I think that was a fork in the road. We started to get it together again.

We planned a few more things, including a skiing trip (something neither of us were into, but it felt good to learn together) and a visit to friends in Lyon for the weekend. As far as trying to start a family was concerned, we knew we needed a strong foundation between us if we were going to go again. We didn't really manage to gather ourselves until late the following spring. We returned to the same clinic, this time for a 'fresh cycle': a full IVF cycle, which would produce new embryos, so that this clinic was in charge of the entire process from start to finish. It was going to be intense. Bootcamp, super-charged.

I started to float the idea at work that this time I'd need to take some sick leave as a chunk of time, as opposed to trying to squeeze appointments in between shifts. I'd been warned that there would be 5 a.m. starts to do injections and then travel into central London to take bloods on a daily basis, so being in or near London was essential, really. Luckily we would have my mum's as a base, nearby.

The plans were underway and the initial preparatory testing began. We had my cytokines tested in May for a cycle that wouldn't happen till the late summer. This was to check the blood to detect those natural killer cells which could kill off the embryo.

I decided to take on a challenge of a different kind at the same time as all this was bubbling up once again. And, although I was sceptical about whether I'd be able to logistically complete it with the cycle looming, I'm so glad I went ahead. With so many other things, I'd said no because of worries about clashes with treatment, but on this occasion I just went for it for some reason – I think because it was a cause close to my heart.

Tori James, the first Welsh woman to climb Everest, had contacted me to ask me to take part in something

4. Rugby full-time, IVF half-time

called The Diamond Challenge, which was being done to mark 60 years of the Duke of Edinburgh's Award. The DofE Award, for which I am an ambassador, is a scheme through which young people can gain bronze, silver or gold awards for personal development through learning new skills, committing to physical activity and volunteering, and finally completing a gruelling outward-bound expedition. I'd completed all my DofE awards at school and university, and it had somehow become part of my DNA. Arguably it was the kind of mindset you nurture on DofE expeditions that had helped me on my fertility journey thus far. Rally round and don't give up. Believe in yourself.

This challenge was to learn to stand-up paddleboard and complete a two-day expedition on the River Wye. So, as I was preparing my body and mind for more hormones and another round of treatment, riding the tides for real helped me stay mindful and in the present. Between SUP practice, I would be taking delivery of and administering pre-cycle drugs such as a medication called Humira. This was designed to help lessen the chance of miscarriage, as I understand it. I even had to have a test for latent tuberculosis to be sure it was safe to use.

In addition to paddling as a distraction, I was also sent to France to cover the latter stages of Euro 2016. Wales were on winning form and we'd reached the finals of the tournament. I found myself back in Lyon again and able to put my fading French into some sort of practice between live outside broadcasts. It felt good being me, doing my job. In those moments, I was in my element. I particularly loved live telly on location. All the juggling seemed worth it.

Looking back at my diary for that period, I think I'd got to the point where I was determined to make the most of things when I knew we *weren't* in a cycle. We had planned ahead and knew when the intense part would start so, for now, I could try to enjoy life. We went to Greece and my family came to stay in Wales in the summer, Lee's sister got married and we caught up with friends. It culminated with me completing my paddleboarding challenge. The weather was against us but we did it by paddling into the night with head torches and I made some friends for life. Just like DofE.

And then September came. Three weeks off. Some space to breathe and focus on the job at hand. And so it began. Day 1 – 14 September 2016. And the first 5 a.m. start to get the train to London from my mum's.

Another – more intense – tutorial for the copious amounts of hormones I'd be injecting every day. More intralipid drips. Every day two blood tests and several self-administered injections, depending on how the follicles which release the eggs were developing on your ovaries, the idea being to get as many follicles as possible ready for the point when they are told to release a mature egg. This routine would continue for 10 days – my stomach gradually getting more and more bruised from injections of Clexane to thin my blood to avoid clotting and assist with blood flow to the womb lining. I realise from some perspectives it may not seem the ideal environment to get pregnant, with body and mind constantly in flight or fight. In some ways, I agree. But there seemed to be no choice. If you've been there, you'll know.

As I pumped myself with more hormones, the follicles grew – and with them, eggs. Every day my tummy would

4. Rugby full-time, IVF half-time

grow larger, more bloated and more uncomfortable. I couldn't zip my jeans up and by the last few days it was very tender and painful to walk. It would certainly be a relief to stop the injections and for the eggs to be removed.

When the time came to administer the trigger injection which would tell the eggs to release, I remember it had to be refrigerated, but after we got it from the clinic we were going back to my mum's for the night. It was only allowed out of the fridge for a certain number of minutes in a cool bag. We reluctantly decided our best chance was just to fork out for a taxi all the way to mum's (about an hour), if we were to be in with a chance of getting it back in time. There was a very precise time (on the minute, almost) that the jab had to be done. The time it took to work would coincide with when they'd booked me in for my egg collection op – the morning after next. So we had this refrigerated box and we were asking the taxi driver to get us home as quickly as he could. I think he thought we had an organ in there, or a finger we'd chopped off. I don't think he thought we were weird – I'm sure he's transported stranger things in his time as a London cabbie.

It all worked out, the injection happened and the eggs were triggered to release. The next step was an even earlier start for the op as I was going under general anaesthetic, so Lee and I had to stay over in a small hotel. In classic Lee style, he had me up and was blaring cheerful music to try to get us in a positive frame of mind. I'm not a morning person at the best of times. He tried.

Lee's sperm donation happened. My egg collection happened. And we waited.

97

Several days actually. The process of fertilisation and survival of the fittest embryos takes about five days. By that time you know which ones are going to reach blastocyst stage (as mentioned before, considered the best stage in the UK to then implant back into the womb). The egg collection was in double figures but when the competition was over, six survived. They would each become our little tiny chances to fall pregnant, along with the few that we had left from France.

Those few weeks of treatment had felt like a year. We had some good embryos from the cycle, though, and all we could hope for was that one of those would be the start of our future family. And whilst most would be frozen for future attempts, the best quality one from this round would be transferred to my womb almost straight away, on 30 September 2016.

So once more, pregnancy test results loomed for us. It was a tense time as usual, though there were still moments to reflect on with amusement. For instance, at this point in the treatment I was prescribed progesterone injections, which had to be kept in the fridge and administered at the same time every evening into my buttock. It was a big needle and an awkward angle to be able to do inject myself, as you can imagine, so, Lee was assigned the job! What followed was that on the days when I was scheduled to work late shifts, he would need to get the medicine from our home fridge (as I did not want that casually stored next to a colleague's sarnies at work!) and then drive to Cardiff to meet me. We would end up either sneaking off into the dressing room with the aforementioned needle, or I'd meet him with his little pouch of drugs in my car in the car park. Neither were

4. Rugby full-time, IVF half-time

a good look and I wonder what my fellow journalists on shift thought we were doing in the dressing room, let alone what might have been caught on the car park's CCTV! We have laughed about it ever since.

During those periods of anxiety, there were always moments like these which brought us smiles. And then often instances of happy tears too. As we embarked on that fortnight of waiting for the test, between injection runs, Lee also gave me a card. As if to try to manifest a positive outcome, it had printed on its front, 'Welcome to planet Earth' and, alongside it he had written, 'Our special gift'.

Chapter 5

Dying to hope

All I could do in those minutes on 14 October 2016 was try to focus on the man who was sweeping the leaves up in that little London park round the corner from the clinic. I still remember the shape of them, their colours. And the small piles growing, along with our anxiety.

The call we were waiting for would be from someone in the admin office who we probably hadn't met before. It would last less than 30 seconds, but would have the power to shatter our world. Again.

I couldn't answer it when it rang, the name of the clinic flashing up on my phone. I made Lee do it. I knew the script. The detached voice would verify our identity and then, clinically, the news would be delivered. I couldn't hear the voice on the other end, but I didn't need to. I knew by his reaction that it was this:

"The HCG levels were less than 5. The blood test was negative."

This was our fifth cycle. Two had been fresh IVF cycles and three were frozen cycles with stored embryos. Add to that the countless cancelled cycles due to my thin womb lining, and you could say we were spent. Emotionally and financially.

By now, we knew very well the depths of doom and despair. But those lows were almost exacerbated by momentarily knowing what relief from this pain felt like. We did, of course, have the one HCG reading above 5 in France, when the levels had kept rising, though in very small increments. I will never quite be able to explain the emotional release I felt when 'something had happened'. Maybe I was pregnant. Just maybe. I remember crying with happiness and relief. Lee felt the same. And I remember, for just a few days, we travelled a little more lightly in our marriage, thinking the baggage of infertility had been taken from us.

But on that park bench, everything was as heavy as lead. How did we get up again from here? Could we manage another leg of this journey?

This treatment cycle had been a big deal. We'd tagged it as our final shot. It was certainly our last shot at making new embryos. I'd taken three weeks off work to be near London and it felt like we had absolutely given it our all. A small circle of people had, by this time, become my confidantes at work and I remember when I let them know that it hadn't worked, I received a really pretty bunch of flowers at the house. I think my sister, Georgina, sent me flowers too. It was all I could manage to get up off the sofa to put them in vases. It felt like someone had died. And I guess they had. The embryo, yes – and with it, hope.

But even when you think hope is no more, it finds a way to reignite. And even when it seems you will never find the strength to go again, you cannot help but be drawn to the flame. There was another card, in the depths of these few weeks, which this time I had I bought for Lee, and its quote somehow became our mantra: 'Proceed as if success is inevitable.'

So once the thickest gloom had lifted a little, we once again had to focus on what might be the next logical move. Please remember, though, that the parameters of logic are skewed when it comes to a fertility struggle. What we saw as perfectly logical, those around us may well have seen as beyond the realms of reason, although I don't think anyone was ever brave enough to say so. After all, most of those who care deeply for you and your plight have never experienced it, haven't got a clue how it feels and can only witness your pain – all the while enjoying the fruits of their own reproduction, which seemed to come so easily. I think they all realised this and they never challenged our personally framed sense of logic, regardless of what they might have been thinking. I'm not sure if this is a good or a bad thing. Probably a good thing, as we wouldn't have listened anyway and would likely have taken offence in the process.

What my logic told me was that we were in October with Christmas fast approaching and that Christmas, by its very nature, is THE worst time of year for anyone with fertility problems. Or that's how it feels. And so we had to reframe it. By reframing it, I mean we had to run away from it. Far away.

I am lucky enough to say that Christmas for me had always been something to look forward to. Growing up, it was a special time of the year. Yes, there might have been the odd domestic disagreement, but overall, I have only good memories of family rituals developed over the years, precious times with relatives and everyone making an extra effort. Now though, since infertility had become an uninvited guest in our lives, Christmas had morphed into a thing of dread for both of us. After

5. Dying to hope

all, Christmas magic begins with children. Year on year since we married, we'd been surrounded by families doing family things, memories being made with the next generation, legacies being moulded. And although deep down somewhere I know that one's legacy on this planet is about far more than having a child, at Christmas it doesn't feel like that. It feels as though having children is all that is worth living for. It's not an exaggeration to say an infertile couple at Christmas simply feel like misfits. And this year, feeling like the freaks would be even harder.

So we ran away. To the other side of the world. To New Zealand.

Believe me, when you are reeling from another IVF failure, the other side of the world doesn't seem too far to go if it means finding friends to spend Christmas with who don't have children either. But at least we were turning a negative into a positive. We tried to forget about the one thing we could never forget about and make the best out of a bad situation.

It felt therapeutic for us to plan for something that would actually happen. It sounds strange to say that, I suppose, in a post-Covid world! Just the idea of a long-distance trip began to drag me up from the depths I had sunk to and helped me tap into what I love – organising, itineraries, places, plans.

It was also going to be therapeutic for Lee on a different level. The first third of the trip – before moving on to visit one of my best friends, who had emigrated to Auckland on the North Island eight years before – would see us visit Jerry Collins' family and Jerry's grave at the south end of the island. The accident had only happened just over a year earlier and although Lee had managed to get over there for his funeral, there was a lot of unresolved grief. Spending some time with Jerry's family could only be healing for him.

December couldn't come quickly enough. We flew into Wellington and headed straight to meet Jerry's sisters. We stayed with them for a few days before we jumped on an internal flight to Auckland, where Lee would be able to see a few more of his rugby circle and we would spend Christmas with my friend Lucy and her husband Neil. I had known Lucy for 15 years, having studied together for our postgraduate diplomas in Broadcast Journalism and started jobs in local television together. She emigrated to New Zealand the same year that I moved to Wales.

To sum up Lucy, she looks amazing and she has an even more amazing soul. A soul that offers just the kind of friendship you need when your mind is in a muddle. She and her husband didn't have children themselves (they had cats) and they knew where we were with trying to be parents. They'd kindly offered to put us up for ten days. An adult Christmas with only fur babies allowed.

We walked on the beaches, visited the best brunch spots and took in the Auckland city vibe. Although there was, without doubt, an underlying tension due to everything we were still processing, it was still proving the right decision to have made. Then on 21 December, one email sent everything off course again. It was from my dad. And little did we know at that moment, but it would change everything.

Now, my dad was a character and we had a unique relationship. I guess that's a stupid thing to say because every parent-child relationship is unique. I suppose I say

5. Dying to hope

it was unique because he lived abroad in Thailand after a divorce from my mum, and over the preceding years we'd had our fallouts over some of his pre- and post-divorce choices, particularly regarding his relationships. But there was still a bond.

I hadn't chatted to my dad for a little while, aside from a couple of messages telling me he'd had an upset stomach and had missed a couple of social engagements. The email in question told me that he'd fallen seriously ill. Now, over the previous few years he'd experienced several health scares. He ended up in hospital in the UK when he collapsed at the airport on his way back to Bangkok and he'd not long told us that he'd been diagnosed with something called IPF (idiopathic pulmonary fibrosis) – a condition which affects the lungs. He'd always been very cautious about all things health-related and often his worries turned out to be unfounded, so when he told us about the IPF, it took me a while to take it in and process it. I was in denial for quite a while, I think, because the forecast is that it could significantly decrease your life expectancy and you're likely to gradually become reliant on extra oxygen to breathe. I'm not sure I'd completely processed it when we travelled to NZ, because I'd had my own medical issues to worry about.

This time, though, he was in hospital again. It was hard to gauge how serious it was and it was hard to get hold of anyone in Bangkok. Then I got another email saying that he would need to have an operation. It turned out none of this was related to the IPF, but it quickly made me all the more conscious that he was not in good general health and whatever *was* wrong, his outlook might be affected by that.

He explained that he had to have an infected abscess removed from his neck and said he'd been told it might already have caused blood poisoning, also known as septicaemia. I didn't know much about it except that it was dangerous. I certainly didn't know how quickly a patient could deteriorate if sepsis was allowed sufficient time to take hold.

Navigating the time difference and language barriers as well as the complicated hospital phone system, I did manage to get through to him on the phone on the ward before the operation. But with his hearing problems and his health, the conversation wasn't very fluid. He told me he was very ill and was scheduled for an operation on Christmas Day.

In hindsight, my reaction was maybe a bit strange, but who knows? Shock is interesting and I think I buried my head – almost literally – in the sand. I headed to the beach with Lee and tried to forget what was happening in a hospital in Bangkok. Then, at the beach, Lee and I had a further mini drama to add to the distraction technique I was embracing. Our hire-car key snapped in the ignition and we were stranded, with ensuing calls to breakdown companies to come to our rescue and to restaurants to find some food at short notice while we were waiting.

Whilst all of that was happening, my dad tried to call me before he went in for his operation and I missed it. He left a voicemail.

The operation was a success in part. They did remove the abscess from his neck, but the infection had already spread and after the surgery he was put into an induced coma to try to aid his recovery. I managed to speak

5. Dying to hope

to the doctor in charge of his treatment and also to a friend of his who was in the medical profession, and they reassured me that he needed to be in a coma to give his body the best chances of fighting the infection, rather than using its limited resources on anything else. That seemed to make sense and I remained optimistic.

Being so far away from my dad and not being able to easily speak to those looking after him, it was very difficult to know what to do next. We were due to fly to the Cook Islands that day and, after a lot of deliberation, I chose to continue the trip, as I felt confident he needed time on strong antibiotics to get better. We'd had a similar situation with a technician at work who had been placed into an induced coma to fight sepsis, and he'd survived and is today fit and healthy. Other than that comparison, I had very little knowledge to call upon.

During our time in the Cook Islands, however, they found some clots on his lungs and my concern started to increase. Then in a matter of days, as we arrived home in the UK, what was already bad turned worse. His insurance company announced they wouldn't cover his treatment. Being a journalist and having covered multiple stories about Brits abroad racking up huge medical bills after accidents on holiday without insurance, I instinctively went into overdrive, speaking to lawyers and the like to try to get advice.

Looking at this in the rearview mirror, I can now see that throwing myself at all the stuff I might be able to control was easier than facing up to my dad's condition. Besides, I actually had no-one to fly out to Thailand with. My parents were friends but divorced, and my mum was 72 – no age to be going through that kind of ordeal for my sake. My sister wasn't able to come for various reasons and Lee had just started a new job, plus we'd been advised by the doctors that, with the prevalence of the Zika virus, which can lead to life-threatening birth defects, Thailand may not be a good destination to expose him to when we were trying to fall pregnant. Either of us could pick up the virus from mosquitoes, but whilst any risk to an embryo if I caught the virus would clear once I'd recovered from the symptoms, less was known about the long-term effects on a man, and the guidance at the time was that it would be six months before it was safe to try to conceive again. On balance, it didn't feel like a good idea. In the end, it was my Aunt Jackie who said she would come, and who was my saviour. I simply would not have coped with the following week without her.

Why am I telling you all of this? Well, because it turned out that message on my voicemail whilst we were dealing with a bust car in New Zealand was the last time I would ever hear him speak to me.

I eventually got to Bangkok and went straight to the hospital, and it was only at that point that the reality of the situation really struck me. He was lying there on a ventilator, connected to what seemed like half a dozen machines. He looked frail, he looked old. His hands and feet were all swollen up with fluid. This was a fit 73-year-old man who still prided himself on going to the gym every day. He would boast about his lean physique and the exercise routine he had always stuck to. When I saw him lying there, I was knocked sideways.

When we returned the following day, I asked if it was possible to bring him out of the induced coma at all, to see if he would come round just a little and recognise

5. Dying to hope

me. They did what I asked but only for a few moments, as anything else would just have been too dangerous for his organs to cope with. I held his hand and tried to tell him I was there and that it was going to be OK. As small as the response was, I do feel (or maybe I simply have to feel) that he knew it was me, that I was there. He was motioning with his hand a little as if wanting to take the ventilator out, but of course that was sustaining his breathing so he couldn't. But the urge was to take it out and to say something. Then as quickly as they brought him round, they said they needed to put him back under. And that was that.

Over the following two days, his condition worsened. My dad's friends in Bangkok started turning up, one by one. And then a vicar I'd sought out at the hospital arrived too. The order of things then is a bit blurred except for these memories. The vicar I think said some prayers round the bed. I've no idea how much time passed between that and what happened next, but then my dad had a cardiac arrest. Everyone was pushed aside but the curtains around the bed remained open and I saw them, from across the room, resuscitating him. Like most people, I'd only seen that on the television.

When they started his heart a second time, I realised I couldn't let him pass like that – for that to be the end. So I spoke to the medics to try to get a definitive picture on what he was facing. In effect, his heart would keep on arresting, they told me. The drugs hadn't worked. His organs were failing him. The sepsis had overcome him. I was then told that to save his heart arresting over and over, his life support could instead be switched off and he could pass more peacefully. It's the hardest decision

I've ever had to make – and on my own, in the space of a few moments. But it was the lesser of two evils.

His friends, my aunt and I were gathered around his bed and the vicar recited the Lord's Prayer. My sister said some words to him via my phone. Then I held my dad's swollen hand and just tried to reassure him, telling him who was there and that we all loved him.

I thought I'd have longer, but it was only a matter of minutes before he went. In a way that comforted me – I knew that I had made the right decision. He was clearly very, very ill and would never have recovered, and it was right to make it stop sooner rather than later.

The next few days were incredibly surreal. My father had left clearly laid-out funeral plans in the event that he died abroad, and had always told me where to find them. I suppose he knew that it was likely I would have to negotiate all of these things on my own. And for this guide, I was very grateful.

My dad's request was that following a more 'British' funeral service, he should be cremated at a Buddhist temple. There is typically a very short space of time in Thailand between death and cremation, so this happened just four days later.

In that space of time, I embraced the Buddhist beliefs regarding death and rebirth and the conviction that a person's spirit remains close in the days after they die. And so I took comfort as close friends came to the apartment to leave his favourite meal for him on the balcony and his favourite tipple (gin and soda). When we went out to eat one evening, an empty chair was left for my dad and food ordered for him. I found it a beautiful show of love and respect.

5. Dying to hope

Following the funeral and temple cremation, I packed up all of my dad's belongings that I could in one suitcase, along with the urn for his ashes, and my aunt and I flew back home. I'd not given myself the chance to let out my grief and when I arrived back at our house in the UK, it was like it surged out of me. It was like nothing I'd ever experienced before. I'd had tasks to complete in Thailand and had had to remain composed and focused to a degree. But now I was in my own space, my mourning was released – and I wailed. I felt it physically in every part of me.

Dealing with the death of my father on top of the failure of fertility treatment, I found very difficult. Only four months before, what we had considered our last chance at a baby had failed in London. And now I'd lost a parent – whose legacy *I* was – it made it all the more poignant that as it stood, I would perhaps leave no legacy of my own. The awareness of my own mortality was intense. Eventually, I turned to medical help and was prescribed sleeping tablets and antidepressants.

But as my grief unfurled itself, we also had to once again focus on what was next for us in trying to be a family. As details of my father's will came to light and over the coming months some of his assets were sold, it became apparent that my dad's passing could have gifted us something incredible. We had ruled out the prospect of using a surrogate: all agencies in the UK had closed their waiting lists due to a shortage of surrogates, which had left us with only the option of going abroad, and only America had reliably sewn up all the tricky legalities that come with asking someone else to carry your child. But for that, you pay. Up until now, the phenomenal US costs had been out of the question for us, but my dad's inheritance could be a game changer. And there was a real chance his legacy could end up being far more than a financial one.

Just like our choice to run away to New Zealand for Christmas, to those around us, running to America may have seemed questionable. And maybe, in hindsight, it was. For we were about to embark on a journey which would not turn out as we had desired or planned. But, like I said, in the realms of all things fertility, hope is a flame that draws you back in.

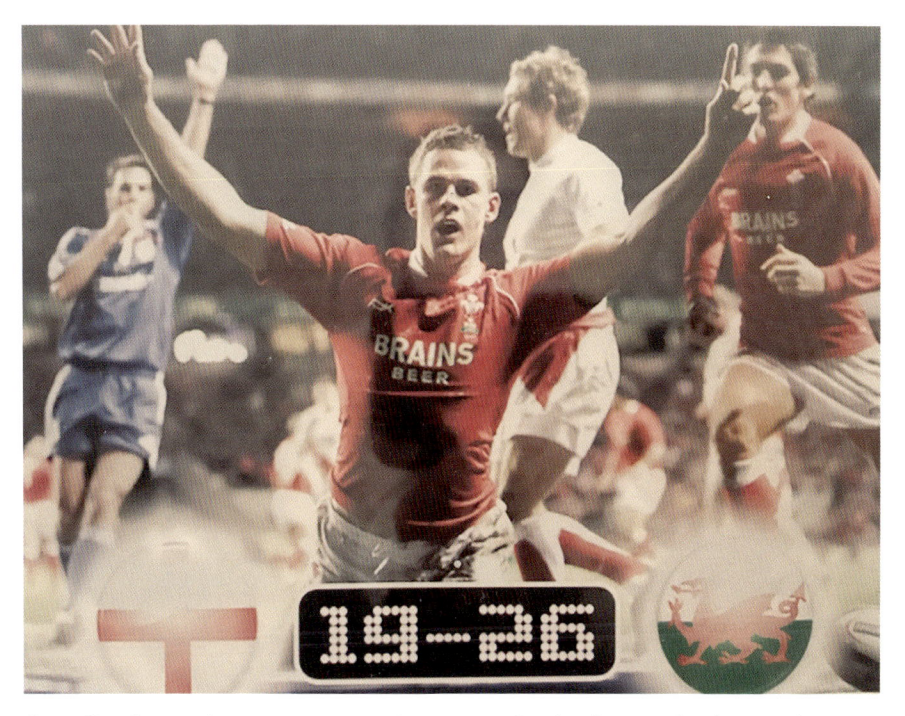

One of Lee's proudest moments, scoring against England at Twickenham in the 2008 Six Nations, not long after I moved to Wales.

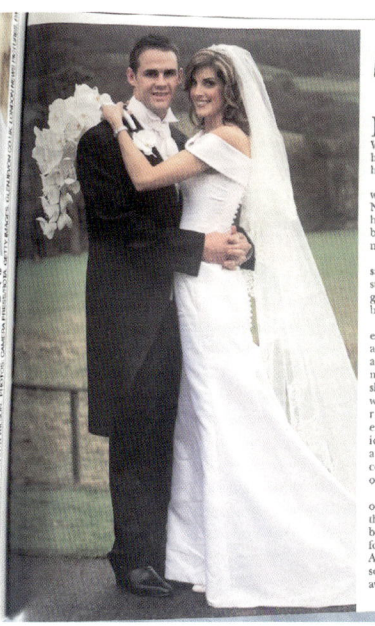

ANDREA BENFIELD MAKES NEWS AS SHE WEDS RUGBY HUNK LEE BYRNE

Beaming as they cut the cake – a tower of delicious brownies – ITV newsreader Andrea Benfield and Welsh rugby union star Lee Byrne couldn't look happier as they celebrate their first moments as husband and wife (below right).

The couple, who got engaged last March after a whirlwind four-month romance, tied the knot on New Year's Day on the Glanusk Estate, in the rolling hills of the Usk Valley in Wales. The estate is owned by the family of Tiggy Legge-Bourke, the former nanny of Princes William and Harry.

"It was simply a dream," said Andrea, who looked stunning in a Suzanne Neville gown and carried a trailing bouquet of orchids.

"We married in the estate's Penmyarth chapel and held our reception in a starlit and candlelit marquee in the grounds," she told HELLO!. Everything was just perfect, from the romantic venue and exquisite flowers to the icing miniatures of Lee and me, which we commissioned for the top of our brownie tower."

The celebrations will go on for a while yet. Following the wedding, it was straight back to training in France for Lee, where he plays for ASM Clermont Auvergne, so a summer honeymoon awaits.

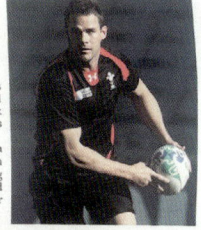

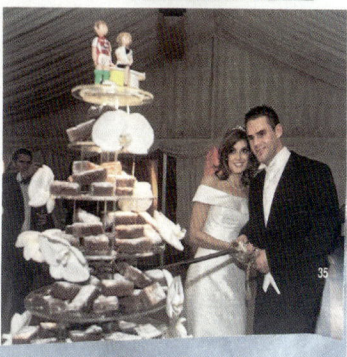

Hello magazine article announcing our marriage.

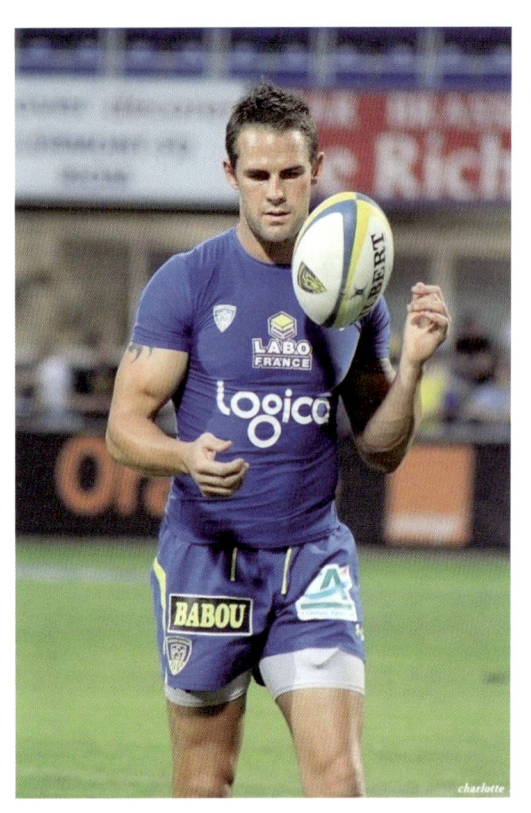

Lee playing for Clermont Auvergne.

Lee in France with our first puppy, Hank.

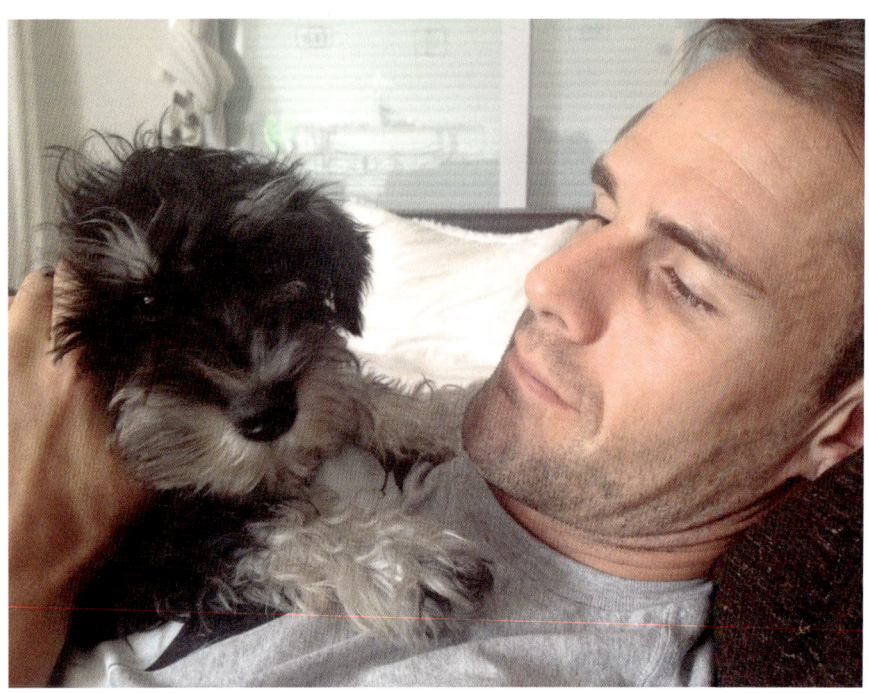

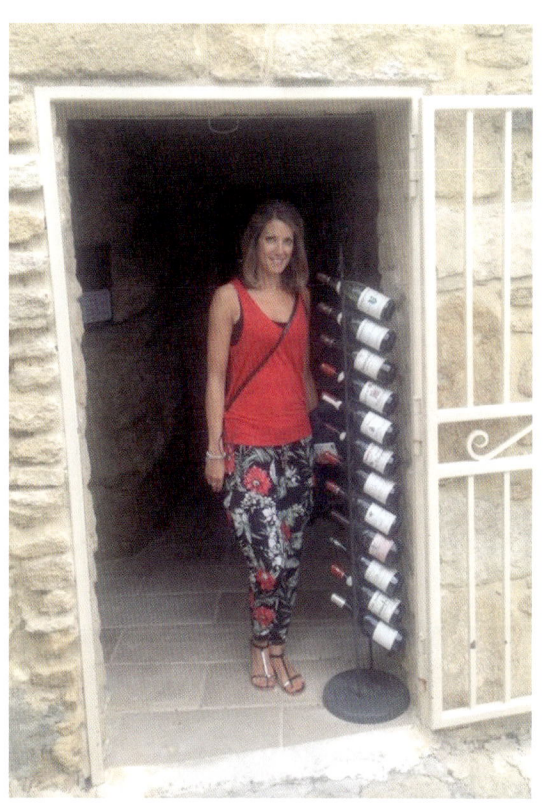

Appearing to be enjoying French culture – in reality, I wasn't even drinking, in order to try to fall pregnant.

Returning from France after unsuccessful treatment, it was back to live outside broadcasts from the NATO conference at Newport's Celtic Manor Resort.

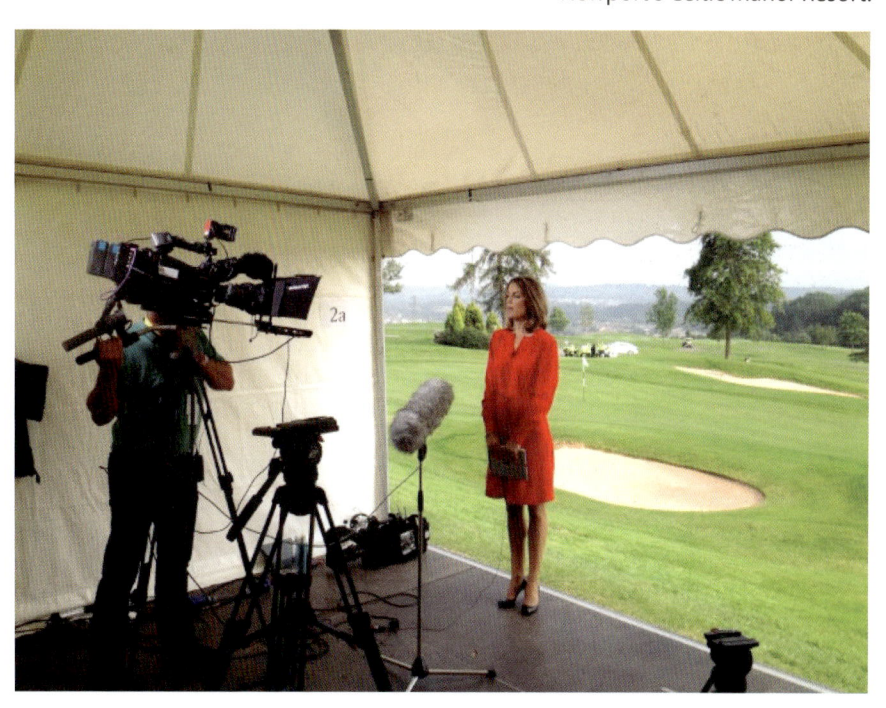

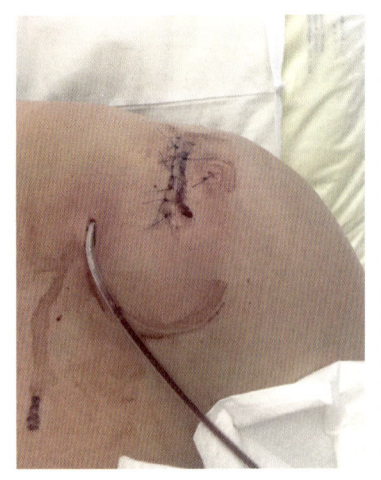

Lee's shoulder after his operation on the injury which ultimately ended his playing career in 2015.

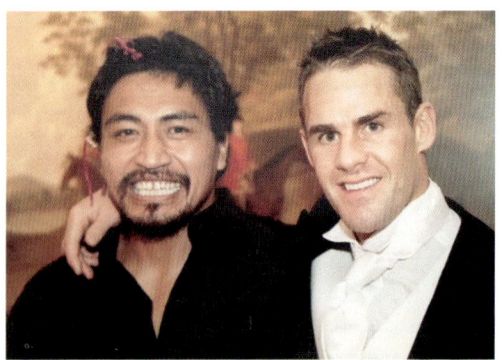

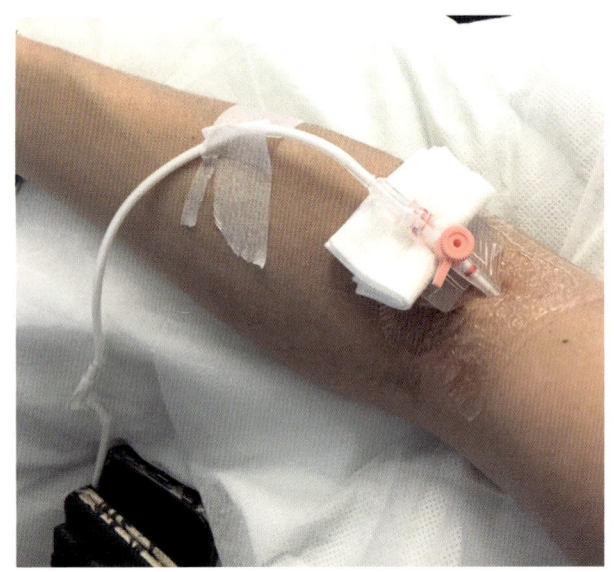

Lee with his close friend, All Blacks legend Jerry Collins, at our wedding – a few years before Jerry died in a car accident.
Glen Jevon photography

My first intralipid infusion at the London clinic, aimed at managing natural killer cells.

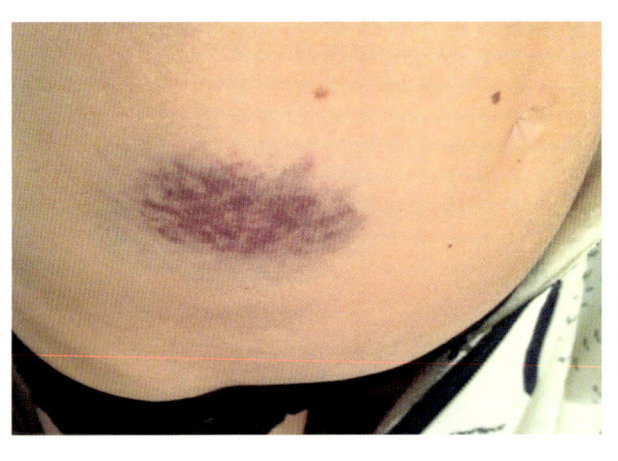

The results of injections in my stomach designed to create better blood flow to the womb, prior to a frozen embryo transfer in London.

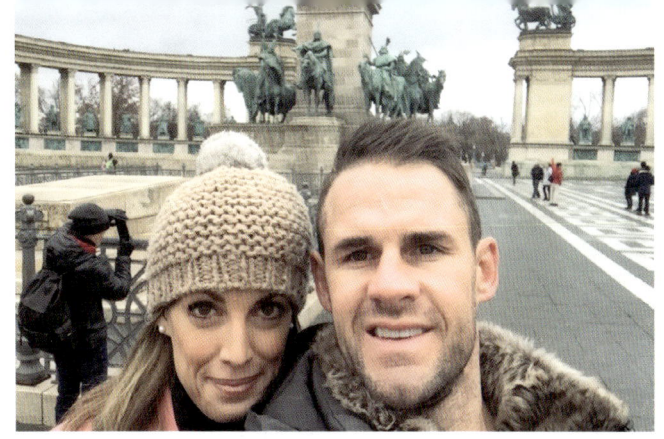

Lee and me in Budapest, rekindling our relationship after we reached rock bottom.

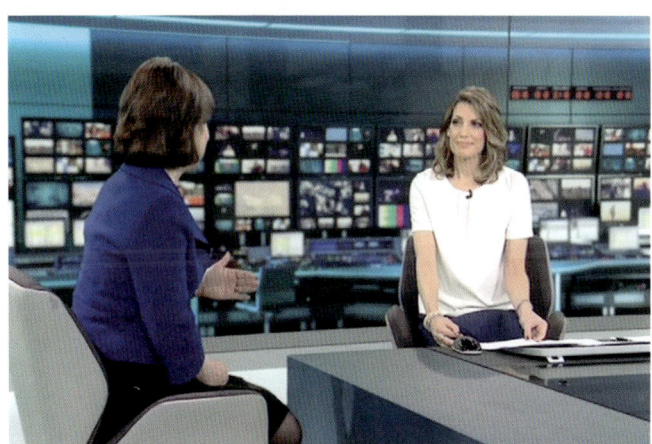

Continuing with my ITN network presentation work between treatment cycles.

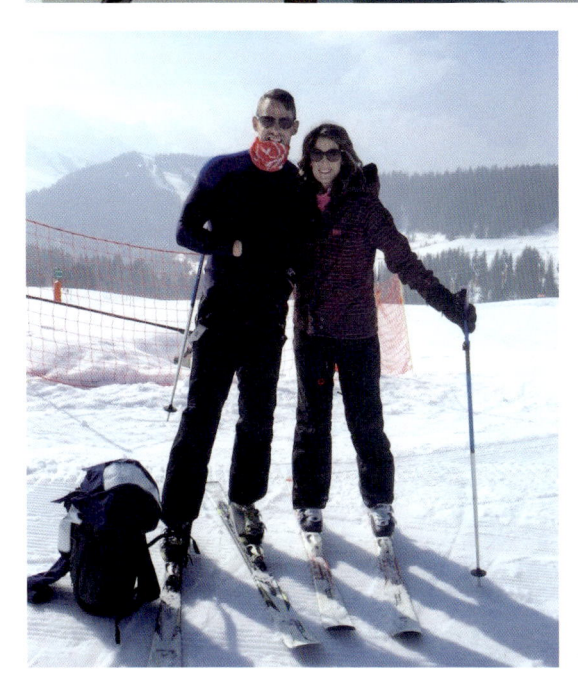

Escaping to La Clusaz, France for our first skiing holiday in 2016.

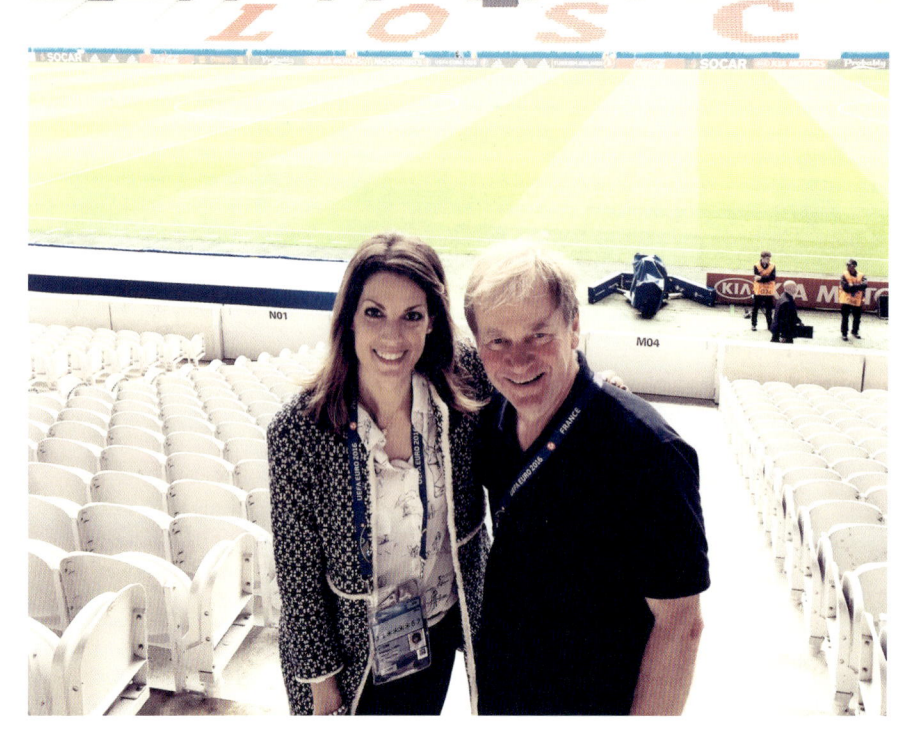

In France with the ITV Wales team (here with cameraman Jerry Cross) to report on the 2016 Euros, prior to embarking on a fresh cycle of IVF.

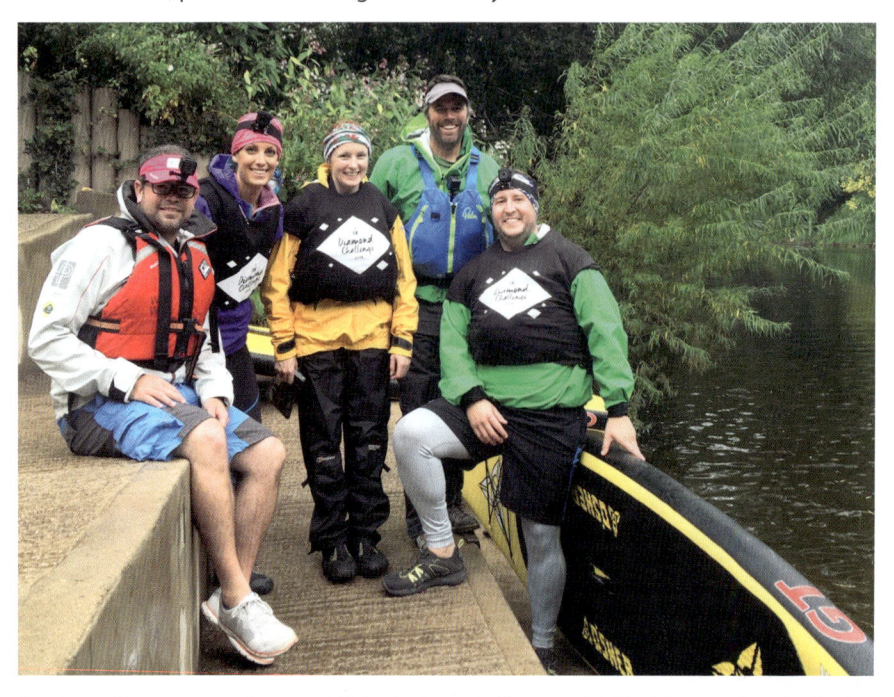

Setting off on my stand-up paddleboarding challenge with Tori James, Simon Clarke, Ben Longhurst and David James.

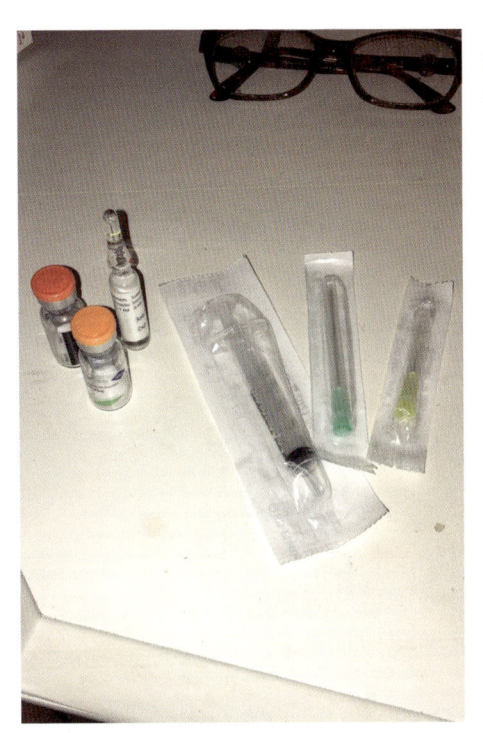

Learning to administer the various drugs as I started a fresh IVF cycle in London.

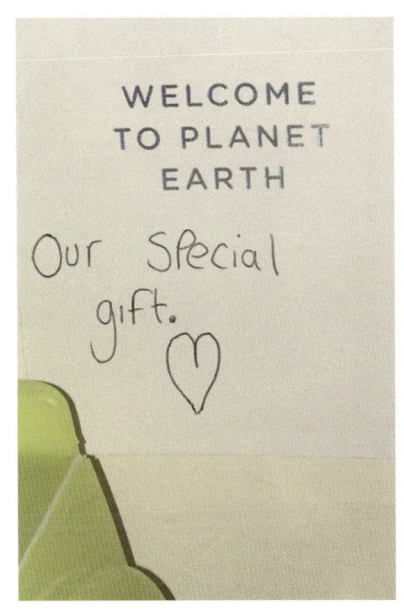

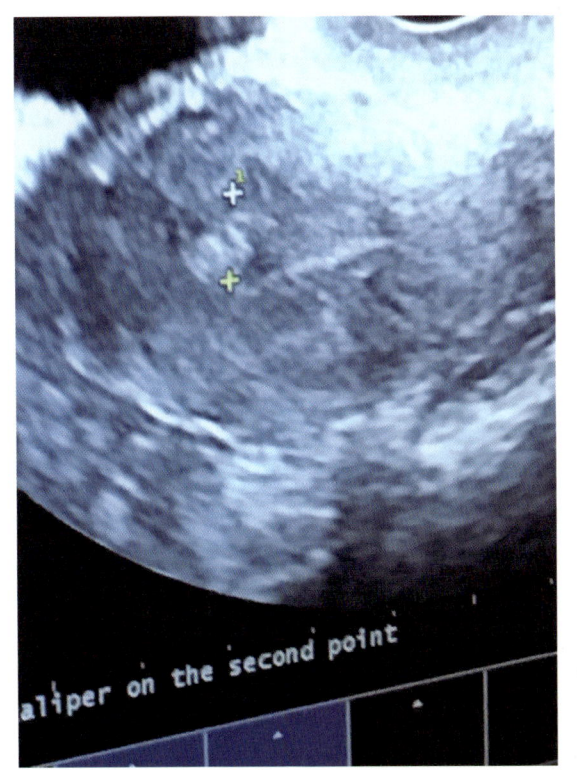

The card Lee gave me as we came to the end of the London IVF treatment and awaited a pregnancy result.

One of the scans measuring my womb lining prior to an embryo transfer.

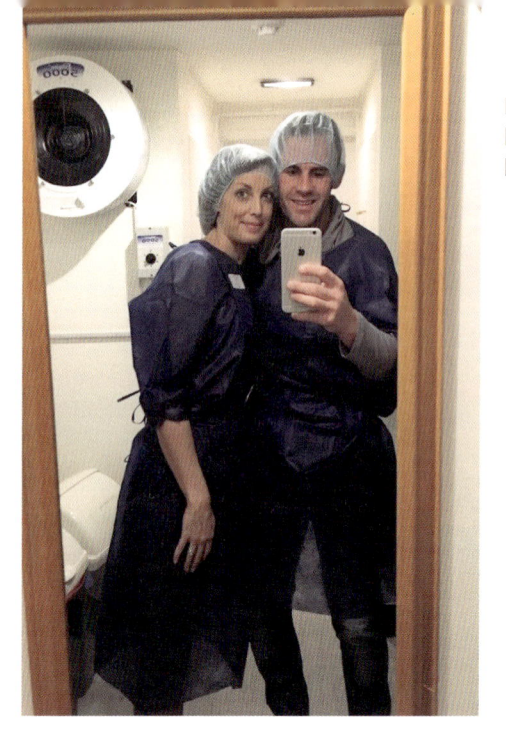

Lee and me immediately before the last fresh embryo transfer we would be able to have.

Lee and me during our escape to New Zealand for Christmas 2016, shortly before news about my dad's critical illness.

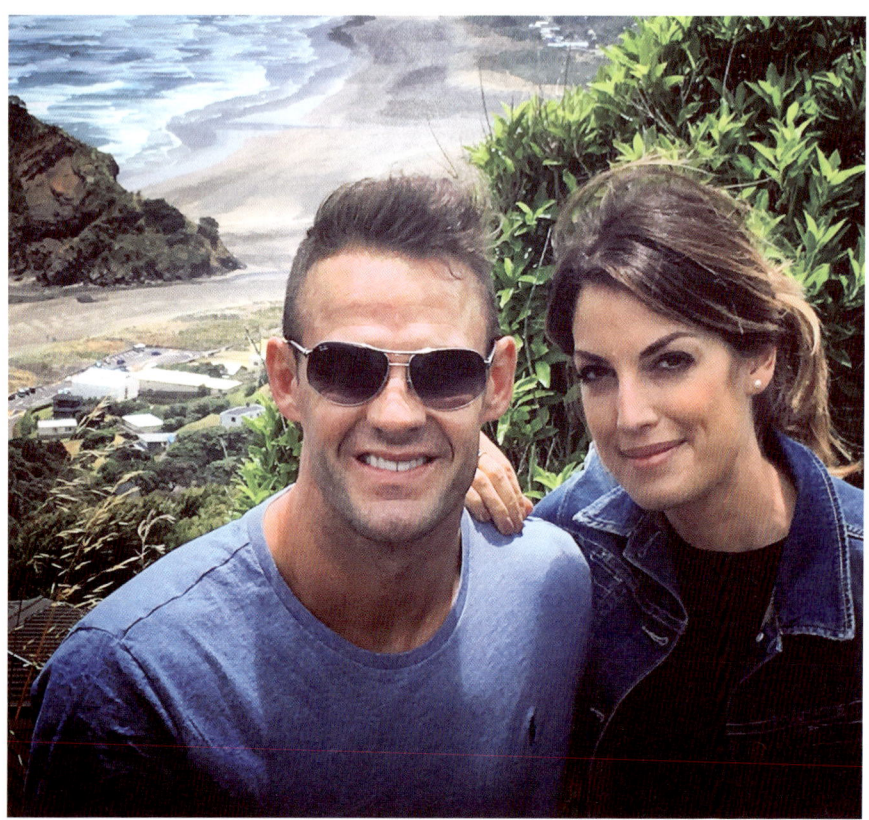

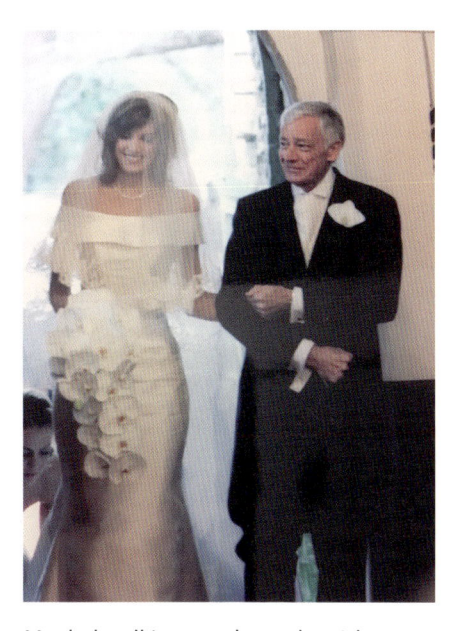

My dad walking me down the aisle at our wedding in 2012.

Glen Jevon photography

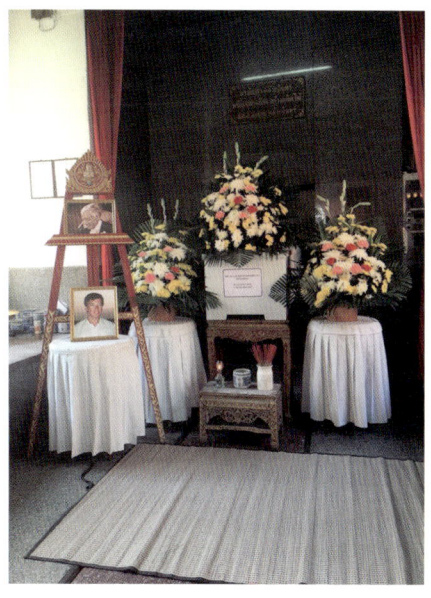

Floral tributes for my dad's funeral and cremation ceremony in Bangkok.

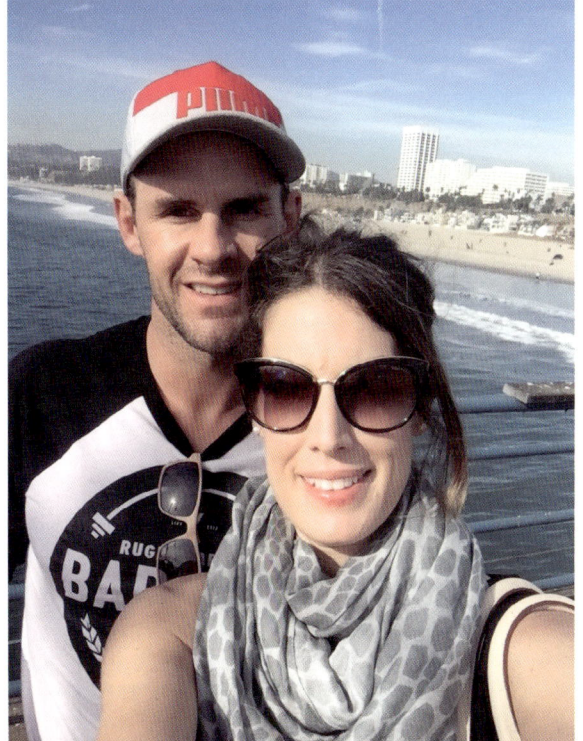

On the famous Santa Monica pier – one of the stops on our impromptu road trip up the west coast of America.

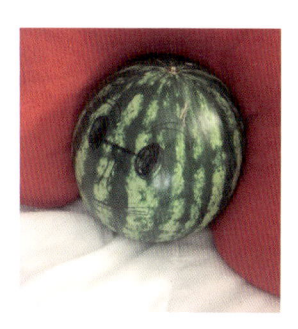

Mary the Melon. A running joke for me and Lee as we tried to stay grounded after the positive pregnancy test in San Diego.

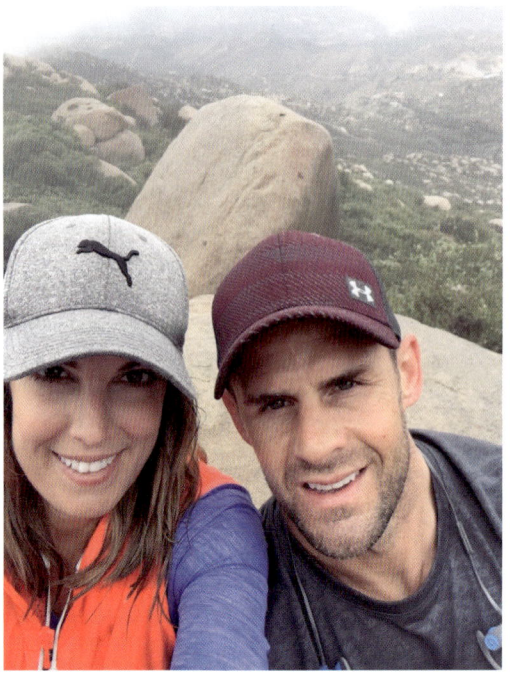

Hiking to stay sane, as we returned to America following the Christmas miscarriage to try again for embryos for a surrogate.

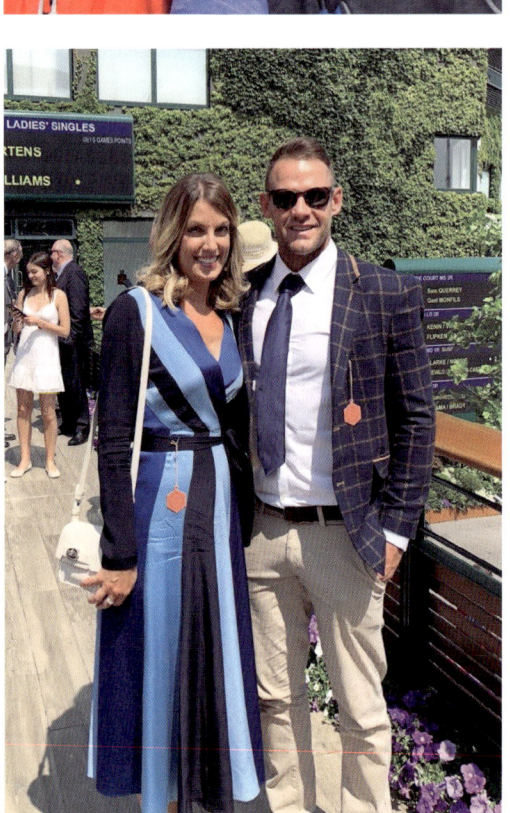

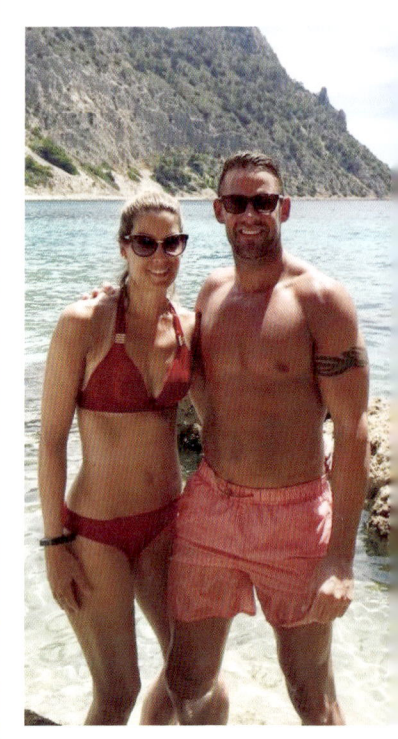

On holiday in Ibiza after being told none of the embryos from the IVF treatment in San Diego were 'normal'. Little did I know when taking this photo, but I was pregnant again.

A few weeks pregnant at Wimbledon, trying to come up with a reason why I wasn't drinking.

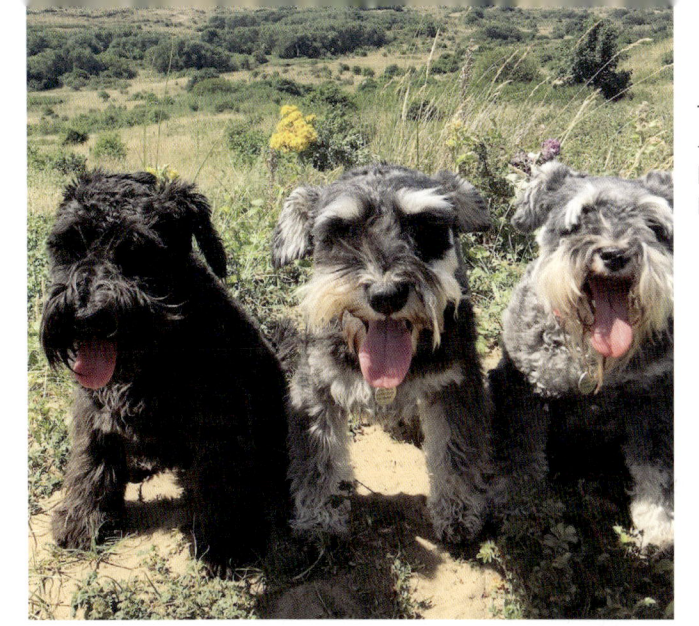

Triple trouble – our three fur babies: Doug, Hank and Marcy.

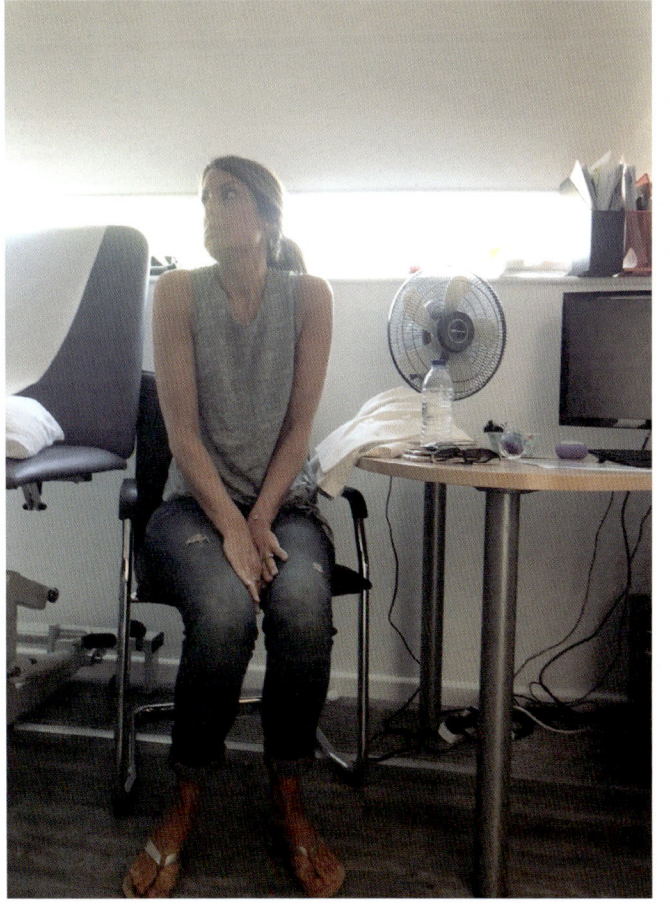

Unknowingly snapped by Lee, waiting for our first scan of Jemima. A few minutes later we heard our baby's heartbeat for the first time.

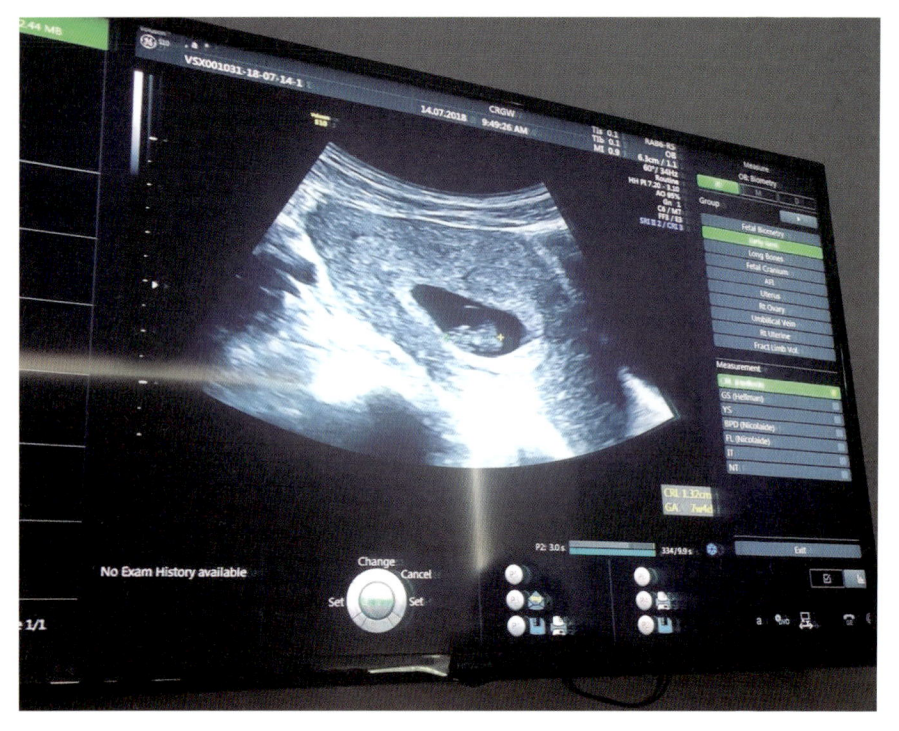

The first scan of Jemima – then called 'Pip'.

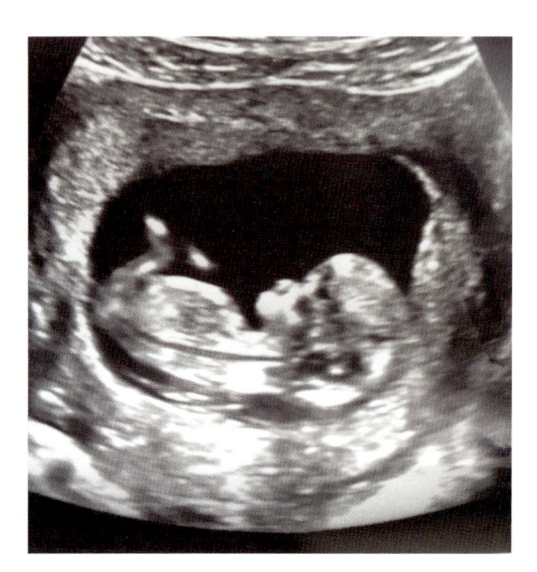

The 12-week scan of Jemima.

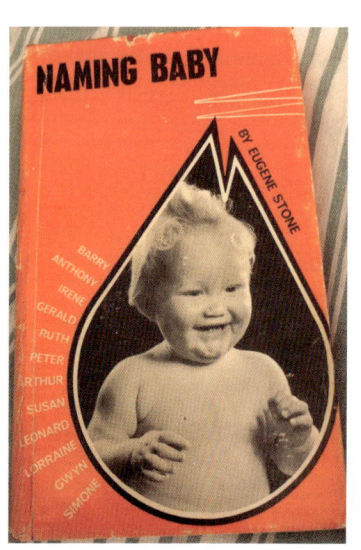

The well-thumbed *Naming Baby* book belonging to my parents, from which I discovered the meaning of Jemima was 'dove'.

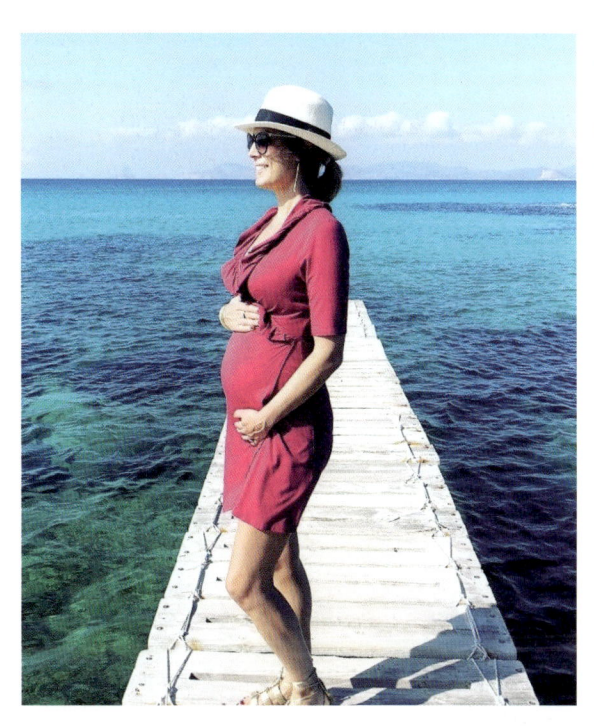

5 months pregnant with Jemima, on Formentera for my 40th birthday. What a gift!

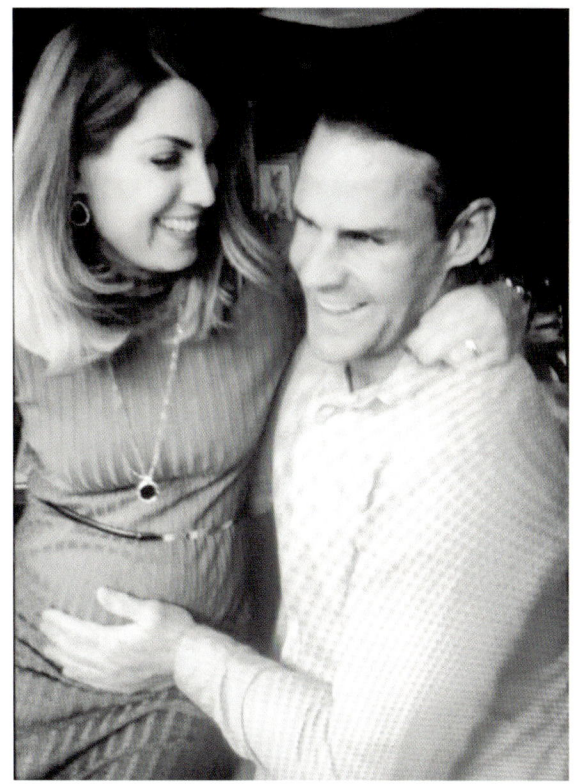

The only photo of Lee holding the bump!

Norman Gregory

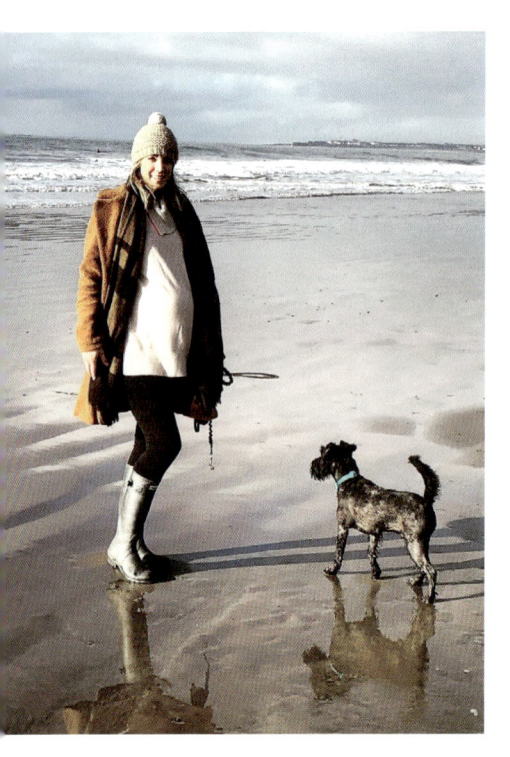

8 months pregnant.

Last day in the ITV Cymru Wales studio, with the bump.

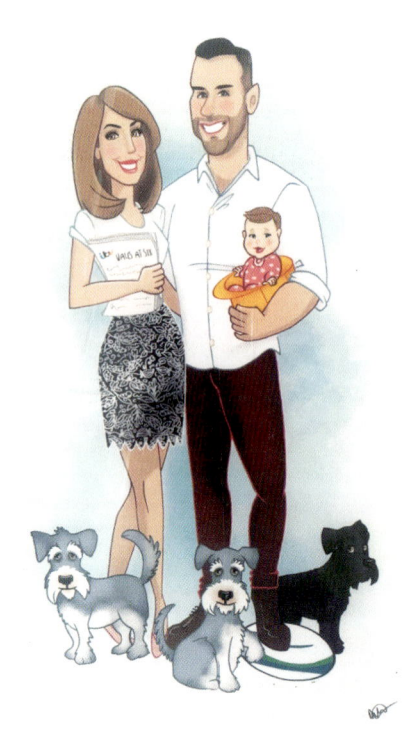

The commissioned art for the nursery wall, featuring the furry and human members of the Byrne family!
Illustration by Alistair Stuart

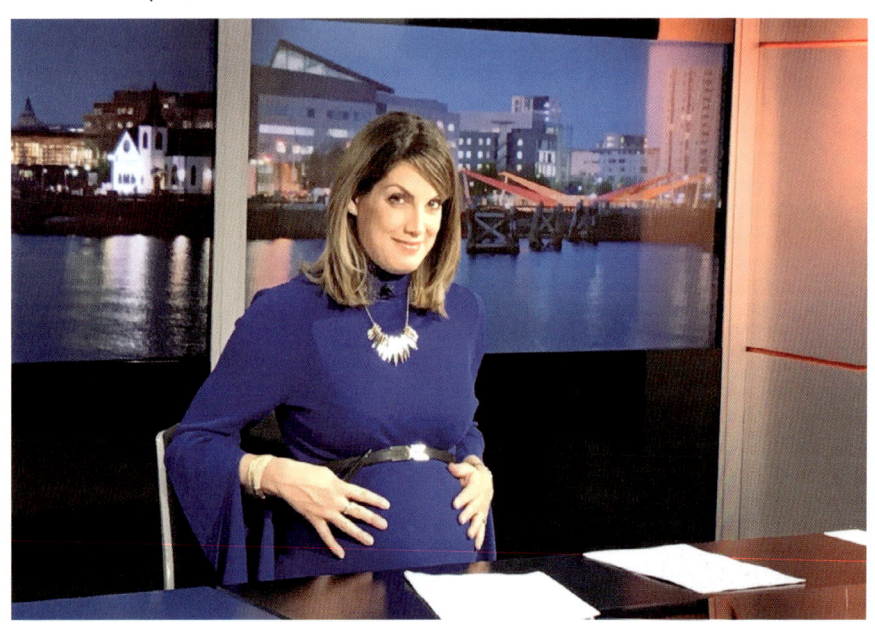

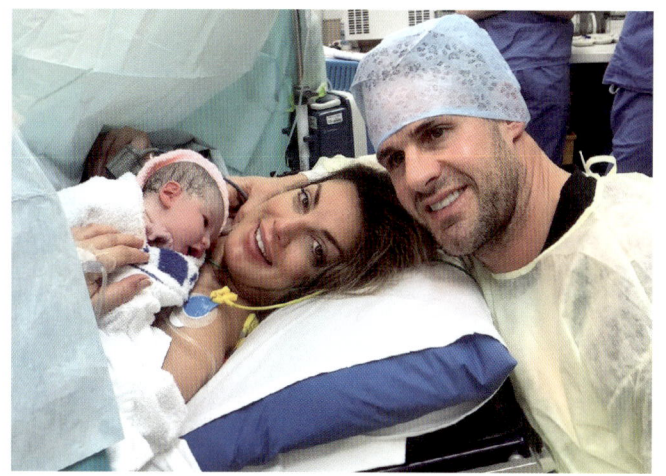

Finally! Our special gift arrives.

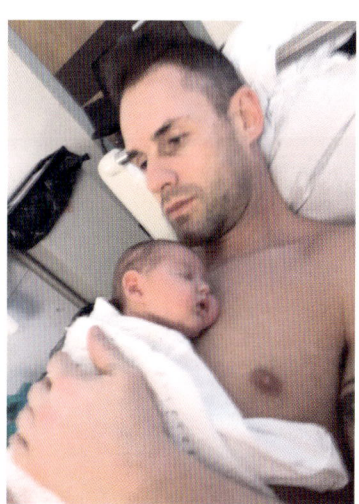

Lee with newborn Jemima.

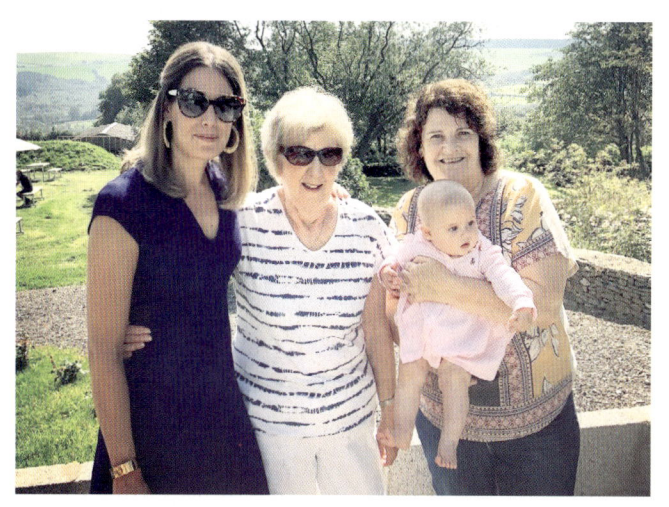

Jemima as a baby, with me and her two grandmas.

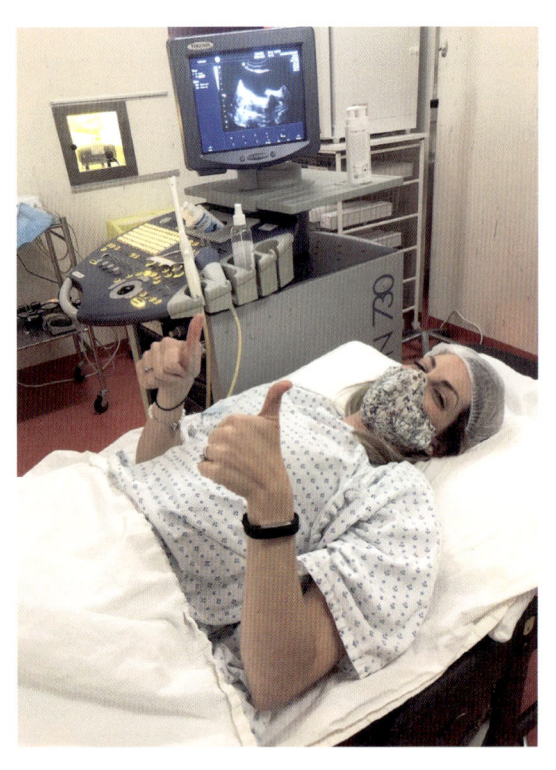

A frozen embryo transfer on my own, due to restrictions at the tail end of the pandemic, to try to make a sibling for Jemima. Sadly, although I fell pregnant, we lost this baby as well.

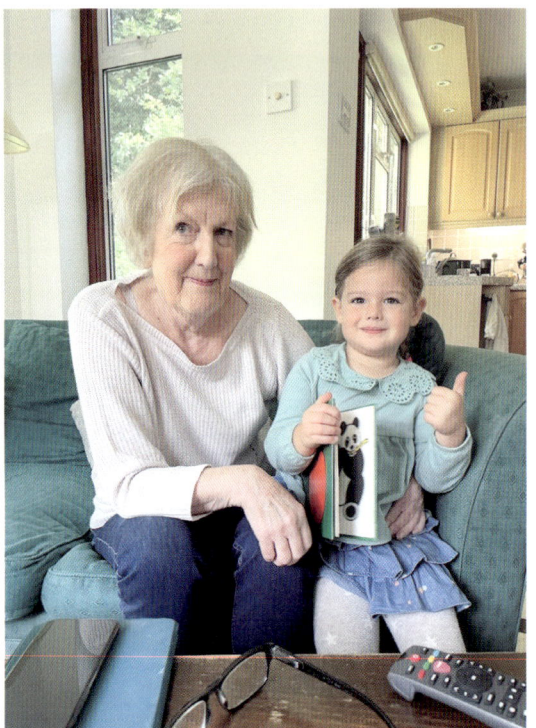

Jemima with Nana (my mum).

CHAPTER 6

The American Dream

AND SO TO America. Over the next few months, we started to explore the options for a Stateside surrogacy plan. It wouldn't be easy and it wasn't how we would ideally have wanted things to go, but it did feel like we had choices and a bit of control once again.

We filled in endless forms and handed over large sums of money just to sign up to the idea. Then we wrote letters to prospective surrogates. Women who had signed up to the agency we were using in San Diego, California, would read the letters and hopefully we would find a match with whom our values and desires for pregnancy and birth aligned. It would be a waiting game.

In the meantime, we needed embryos to be able to transfer to a surrogate and all the advice stated that we should create these at a local clinic in the USA, rather than use the embryos we had created in London or in France. The guidelines followed in America at the time said that all embryos should be genetically tested for abnormalities, and this would be done in the developmental process in the lab.

Our doctor, I had already decided, was some kind of angel. In the first video call we had with obstetrician-gynaecologist Sandy Chuan, she was sitting in her office in a chair with a large feathery white cardigan over the back of it. The way the light silhouetted it made her look heavenly and I took this as an omen for our treatment. Though 'sent from God' may have been a little far-fetched, she was lovely. And these comparisons were maybe one way of alleviating the pain of how much money it cost to be seen by her.

Once again it was a tricky juggle of dates and work, but we planned to go to San Diego for an IVF cycle in November 2017. As Sandy also explained, there would (as usual) be some pre-treatment before the main slog of the cycle itself. Depending on the drugs protocol each clinic decided to put me on, there was always medication to take in advance. This time I remember it being some kind of inhaler that would be part of switching off my body's normal cycle, so our doctor could take it over and control what my hormones did and when.

I was, as usual, working right up to departure and the day before we left, I hosted one of Wales' biggest awards ceremonies – The Nurse of The Year Awards. My hormones were going haywire at this point but I'm hoping the make-up and the cocktail dress belied my tiredness and angst.

Beneath the ongoing work demands, I was terrified of getting the timing wrong with the drugs and ruining the whole plan. Flights, hotels and appointments were booked and it felt like a lot was depending on me following things to the letter and my body playing its part and responding correctly. I remember getting on the plane and feeling relief that we'd got that far with the specified schedule.

We flew to LA and stayed overnight in a hotel by the airport, then picked up our hire car and began our journey

6. The American Dream

to San Diego. We were staying in a hotel apartment, near downtown. It meant we had hotel facilities, but also a little kitchenette so we didn't spend even more of a fortune on food.

There were a few days of acclimatising and finishing off the pre-treatment. Then we had our first appointment at the clinic, where they would do the baseline checks to make sure my body was where it should be in the manufactured cycle. They check your womb with an ultrasound to make sure the lining is thin – which it should be at the start of treatment. And then they do a blood test to make sure your hormone levels are also on track, to enable them to then build from there over the next two weeks with the injections which would stimulate my ovaries.

I had the scan and there wasn't anything out of the ordinary to be seen. I had the blood test. And we went away with the medication we needed to start the treatment.

The next day or so not much needed to be done. We got groceries in for the next week, knowing this hotel apartment would be our home for a while, but also made a plan to treat ourselves to a meal out the next day for Thanksgiving. We went for a meal at a beautiful hotel resort and sat in the sun contemplating the next few weeks, trying to relax. Until, on the way home, we somehow managed to completely run out of petrol. I say 'somehow' to be generous to my dear husband. He had, very kindly, been doing all the driving but hadn't noticed the warning light which had come on sometime previously. I thought he was winding me up when he juddered across three lanes of the highway and we ended up sitting in our hire car, pulled over on the hard shoulder on a public holiday!

Cue only the second time in my life, I think, that I've hitchhiked (which I would not recommend, but at least both times I was with a man). The first time was on a long walk back from an idyllic but isolated beach in Lanzarote when my friend Carl and I were picked up by an old couple pootling their way back to their resort. I'm not sure we even thumbed them – I think they just saw us and felt sorry for us. This time all I can recall is starting to clamber up the side of the US highway and opening Google Maps to find out where the nearest gas station was, when a car pulled over and came to a stop in front of us. It was a lovely, bubbly, friendly middle-aged lady on her way to see family and she took us to fill up a can of gas, before also dropping us back at our car. There is kindness in the world. Maybe it actually turned out in our favour that it was a holiday. More likely to get the sympathy vote, I suppose.

The experience had slightly taken the shine off our special holiday lunch, but in the end it did provide a distraction from the wait for the clinic to call to tell us that I'd taken all the drugs at the right time and they'd had the desired effect, so we were OK to start the treatment proper as planned.

The next day, *with* a full tank of petrol, we took a road trip in the other direction, to a nearby upmarket beachside town called La Jolla (pronounced 'La Hoy-a'). I'd read about it in my pre-trip planning and it looked like a cute place with boutique shopping and nice eateries. We spent the day, once again, trying to take our minds off things. I bought shoes (what better way to distract me?)

6. The American Dream

and we went to the beach. There's even a photograph of me sitting on a towel pretending to meditate. There really was a feeling of positivity. We were here and we were getting something done. The journey to having a family was, at least, moving on again.

Shoes loaded in the trunk and zen state of mind partially accomplished, we started to make our way back to the hotel-apartment downtown. That was when we got the call from the clinic. I saw the number and I answered straight away to get the results we needed to make the next lot of appointments.

The nurse on the other end then said something totally unexpected. I don't remember the exact words, but she told me I was already pregnant. Naturally. Before the treatment cycle had even started.

I must have repeated the words because Lee swerved the car and pulled it to an abrupt stop. I kept asking her if she was sure, and how this could be? And what do we do now? I had never been in such disbelief about anything. Our heads were both spinning. We were giddy with incredulity.

She explained that we could have a repeat blood test to check the HCG levels were doubling in the way that they should to indicate a viable pregnancy, but it was too early to see anything on an ultrasound scan. We went back for a repeat and the hormone levels of human chorionic gonadotropin had risen accordingly. As you'll recall, they are meant to double every two days to show things are developing in some way.

It was a strange time. We were in a strange city. A few days before I had done an unexpectedly strenuous and twisty yoga session (minus orange pants!) with the theory that once I started the IVF drugs and the follicles began growing, I'd not be able to get on a mat for a while. I immediately began to worry that the shapes I'd forced my body into would not have been suitable for a tiny embryo trying its best to stick where it needed to in what was meant to be a pretty hostile womb environment, by all previous medical accounts.

Apart from worrying, there was going to be little more we could do in San Diego. From this moment on, it was a case of keeping the faith. It would, in fact, be weeks before anything could be confirmed on a scan. But we did have three weeks' annual leave booked. I think we spent the next few days going slightly out of our minds. To give you an example, we had all this food we'd bought in the apartment, including a watermelon. One day, I came back from a walk and for some reason Lee had drawn a face on the melon and put it in a red neck rest – the type you use on aeroplanes. We even named it Mary the Melon. It reminded me of the volleyball called Wilson in the film *Castaway* with Tom Hanks. Mary became a way of finding humour to deal with what had become a surreal situation and Lee kept making jokes about how well we were looking after Mary. I also remember hearing the song 'Feel It Still' by Portugal The Man playing over and over on a man's radio outside a bar in town, and I can't hear that song now without thinking of looking after Mary the Melon and how she'd become a metaphor for what my own body was trying to nurture.

To that soundtrack, we decided that as we had the time off, we'd budgeted for treatment (albeit with credit!), and we had a car, why not go and see the west coast of America, take the opportunity to relax as much as we

6. The American Dream

could, and do our best for 'Mary'? And so we checked out of our hotel, made a vague plan to hit certain towns and cities en route in the time we had and took to the road.

We created a whistlestop tour which took us up along California's coast from San Diego to San Francisco. We rode the big wheel on Santa Monica Pier, spent a chilled night in Santa Barbara, visited Bubblegum Alley in San Luis Obispo, saw the places where TV's *Big Little Lies* was filmed in Monterey and bought a picture for our baby's nursery (yes... our baby!) in San Jose, before ending up in San Francisco for a slightly longer stop. There we were able to take in Alcatraz, the Golden Gate Bridge and soak up the Christmas build-up in the city. It went by in a flash, but we were incredibly grateful for the position we were in and for the opportunity to do it, however brief. Before we knew it, it was time to drop off the car and catch a flight back to Los Angeles, to fly home to London.

In the airport, I remember analysing over and over how I was feeling. Each and every twinge. Were they a good sign or a bad sign? What did the bloating mean? How was I meant to feel? And that was the problem, of course: I had no idea. Up until now, I truly had convinced myself that my body didn't know how to fall pregnant. So I was anxious. The theme music to that trip continued to be vivid. I remember 'Runnin' (Lose it All)' featuring Beyoncé playing repeatedly in the airport complex as we waited for our gate. I was too scared to believe in what my body was apparently doing, and also too scared not to. We could not afford to lose it all.

The plane journey home was another few hours of worrying. Ideally, they don't recommend flying until the

119

second trimester, so until 12 weeks, but what choice did we have? We needed to get home and most people at this stage wouldn't even know they were pregnant. It was only due to our very specific circumstances that we'd found out right away.

Even when we landed, the worry didn't end. I readjusted over the next few days to the fact that I would not be free of this anxiety for another few weeks – until we could have an early reassurance scan which would actually show us something was growing in there. Those were some of the hardest weeks. We would veer from venturing into talking about baby names, to checking ourselves and reining in the optimism. It was enough to send anyone loopy. Constantly checking your own thoughts and autocorrecting your positivity before you press send to your vocal cords. We both knew how sensitive we were at that moment, and it was very easy to say the wrong thing.

The weeks ticked by slowly until we got to 8. When your period's late, it's 4 weeks since your last period, so it's said at that point that you're 4 weeks pregnant. So after we'd done a couple of weeks of travelling, there were probably a couple more to go before we could scan around mid December – though it felt like an eternity.

I remember very little about the day of the scan. We were booked in with Dr Amanda O'Leary, who had overseen our Tamoxifen prescription previously and had become our trusted doctor close to home. She was the consultant at the clinic near Cardiff which our French embryos had now been moved to from London – as well as the remaining embryos we created in London. She was lovely beyond belief. Always treated you as an individual

6. The American Dream

and not a number on a file, always found the time to email – at any time of the day or night. A true rarity in this fertility game, where you feel much of the time as if you're on a drugs and appointment conveyor belt.

We arrived, waited and went in. She said, "I know how you're feeling. You really do want me to scan you. But at the same time, you really don't." She just got it. I want you to scan me if you are going to keep our dream alive. I don't want you to scan me if you are going to shatter our world.

I lay down and got myself ready. Lee was quiet. We both were. We were on tenterhooks. What was happening in there with that tiny embryo? With our baby?

Dr O'Leary did her thing with the vaginal ultrasound scanner so she could see the image of the inside of my womb appear on the screen. With carefully chosen words, she said, "I can see a little baby. There they are."

And then something like, "I can't find a heartbeat. The baby is measuring quite small. But that could be because your dates aren't what you think they are."

My head was whirring. I was spinning out. I was thinking the worst. Amanda kept speaking. I was hearing but not processing. She said she would print out the scan pictures of the tiny little baby and we should come back in a week to see how they had grown and if a heartbeat could be found.

We went away and sat silent in the car for a good while, until realising we were on two different ends of the emotional spectrum with this. I had listened to the numbers that Amanda had measured and, going on the results of my googling in the run-up to this appointment, I'd already decided that returning for a scan was just a formality. That really it was already known that the tiny little baby had stopped growing. Everything I read suggested the same. A patient gets asked to come back in a week so they can make sure. But usually, making sure meant confirming the worst.

Lee, on the other hand, remained positive – what I regarded as blindly optimistic. He said I was being negative and that we did not know it was bad news, that we needed to remain in a good frame of mind. That I needed my body to remain in a strong place. It was agonising to not be on the same page. I felt that for my own sanity, I needed to accept what had happened and not hope any longer than was sensible. But Lee still had hopes for my body, for our baby. How could I keep dashing them?

I was at work all of that next week and it was one of the hardest of my life, without a doubt. I did tell my boss that it had looked like we were pregnant, but we weren't sure if we were any more and I might need some time.

The following Saturday we returned to the clinic and to Amanda. By now, I knew the drill. To a degree, I had prepared myself, though I'm not sure Lee had.

She scanned. There was a tiny little baby there still, but you could see it was now even smaller and sort of shrivelled up. That's the only way I can describe it and I knew before she said it that there was no heartbeat to be found.

And that was that. The American Dream – shattered. And with it we gained official membership to a club no one wants to join: the pregnancy-loss club. We had thought we'd lost an early chemical pregnancy in France, but this was indescribably worse.

6. The American Dream

I'll be honest: all I really understood of miscarriage up to that point was what I'd seen on television. A woman is pregnant. She has a bleed. She's no longer pregnant. Simple. It's portrayed as nothing more than an unexpected menstruation. Over within moments.

Let me tell you, this is not the case. It varies incredibly from person to person, but no miscarriage is a little bleed over in minutes. The appointment I described when it was confirmed there was no heartbeat was shortly before the Christmas break. Part of me thought that maybe this could at least all be over by the 25th itself. One small consolation. Little did I know the hoops we still had to jump through.

What I'd had was a missed miscarriage. This is when the heartbeat has stopped and that has been 'missed'. In other words, you don't miscarry and bleed when the heart stops beating, when life is extinguished. Your body doesn't realise at that moment that it should start to let go. It clings on, although there's nothing to cling on to. In our case it was a scan that revealed there was no longer life there, but often it can be that it's a few weeks after the baby dies that your body will finally begin to bleed and shed the products of pregnancy – which in itself is a terribly clinical phrase. This was our baby, after all, not merely a medical process.

We were referred to the Early Pregnancy Unit, which is where you go to get checked out if you feel something is wrong in the first two trimesters of pregnancy. It's the same place women will be sent to get positive confirmation of a pregnancy and it's also yards away from the maternity unit, where people are leaving with their newborns and relatives are coming in to deliver good wishes. We knew we were going in to have bad news confirmed, but we had to go through the scan again before they could decide on the best management. Excruciating.

There were choices. We could have a D&C (dilation and curettage), which was to have the baby removed from the womb through an operation; we could have 'medical management', where drugs would trigger the body to begin bleeding and get rid of the baby itself; we could do nothing and let it happen naturally.

I was adamant I didn't want an op, as I was totally paranoid about how that could affect my lining. And I didn't want to leave things to chance and wait and wait for as long as it might take. So, we opted for medical management. This was right before Christmas now and I remember being given the choice that we could take tablets orally, or we could have drugs administered vaginally. We didn't really want to hang around any longer than we had to, listening to newborn babies cry as we were losing ours, so we opted for the tablets by mouth because we would have had to wait for a more senior medic to become available for the vaginal administration, and they were busy delivering actual babies.

We took the pills and we went home. And we waited.
And we waited. And we waited.
Nothing.
And this took us to Christmas Eve. When there seemed to be no one to speak to and no one to make sense of things for us.

We would go through Christmas in limbo. I'd never known mental anguish like it. Being pregnant, but not pregnant. If that makes any sense. And to make it worse,

6. The American Dream

we were hosting that Christmas and we were meant to have family around, one of whom I'd been told was set to announce a pregnancy. Well, there was no way I was going to be able to hold it together if that happened. An undercooked turkey, burnt roast potatoes or someone forgetting the brandy sauce was one thing. Expecting me to cheer for a pregnancy announcement at this point was quite another. I had to cancel things. I hope it goes without saying that I thought the pregnancy news was fantastic for them and I know they would not have intended to cause us any distress, but it was all just too painful for me at that moment. I'm not sure what Lee might have told them when cancelling, or how much they already knew, but either way I hope they understood.

Christmas came and went. I cooked, we ate, we played games, we had a drink. I smiled, I laughed, I hosted a smaller gathering of just some immediate family. It was as though we put all our feelings and our reality on pause. Then on Boxing Day, it flooded back in. We were back on the phone and we were back to the pregnancy unit to try to make sense of everything.

It turned out that the oral tablets had not been the best proposal. They didn't seem surprised in the least that they hadn't worked. This time, we were put in a side room to wait until someone was free from baby duty, left to listen to those little cries again from the maternity ward, and eventually saw a doctor who was able to administer the vaginal drugs.

Home we went again to wait.

This time it happened as predicted. I hadn't known exactly what to expect. But it was horrific and came in waves of agony, like what I imagined contractions might feel like. It culminated with the loss of the pregnancy. That feels like a throwaway summary of what happened, but without going into too much detail, I could see, as well as feel, that I was losing the beginning of a very tiny baby and that will always stay with me.

The bleeding continued for a long time after that, like a very long and heavy period. And my body continued to look and feel pregnant for even longer. My breasts were heavy and sore and my stomach was swollen. To feel like I was still pregnant, but not be pregnant, really was impossibly hard.

Even harder is that no one really talks about miscarriage. It's awkward. It's taboo. There's a stigma attached. It involves death, grief, physical pain and mental anguish, so I do get why. But one in four pregnancies ends in a loss, and too many people who want to talk and be supported end up suffering in silence. Well, I see you, and I hope the more we do talk, the less torment we will all bear.

CHAPTER 7

The club

I DON'T REALLY know how, but by spring, we had bounced back. Becoming a familiar line, isn't it? We'd decided we were ready to go again to America. This may have seemed like a fool's errand to many, but I couldn't let the chance pass me by. At that point I wasn't ready to accept that it was game over. I'm not sure how Lee felt. He may have been letting me do what I needed to do. But what I do know is that we were both equally stubborn, and his competitive instinct to keep playing your best game until the final whistle meant that he would not give up on Project Baby easily either. He wanted a win more than at any time in his sporting career.

We went through the same build-up to the treatment and we travelled over once again to San Diego, trying to put aside the terrible loss we'd had at Christmas time, and trying even to put a positive spin on it. Although 'at least you know you can get pregnant' is on my list of phrases you absolutely should not say to someone who has lost a baby, between the two of us it was in a small way useful to acknowledge that we had at least started to grow a tiny baby. Painful progress.

The treatment cycle went ahead as planned this time around. You know the drill by now: I had a lot of drugs, got very bloated as my many follicles grew, and then had a small op to retrieve the eggs that had matured. I had a good number of eggs and after an agonising few days' wait, we were told they had managed to develop into a good number of embryos. We made our way back to Wales and back to work.

But there was one big final hurdle to overcome, and that was chromosome tests for any suspected abnormalities. It wouldn't be possible to implant any embryo into a surrogate in America unless these tests were clear.

On 21 May 2018, we were standing at the edge of a new future. Ready to take the leap into the unknown. Ready to have someone carry our baby. Ready to embrace all the logistics, politics, pressure and costs which would come with that. All so we could embrace a new life. Hold it in our arms. Be a family.

But it wasn't meant to be. As you will have read in the Prologue to this book, not one embryo was clear of suspected chromosomal abnormalities. None were 'viable'. There would be no surrogate unless we tried again with another round of IVF in the States. The miscarriage and now this meant this time around things felt irretrievable. We tried to cling on, but gradually we realised that the costs were now spiralling out of our grasp. Not only had the surrogate agency costs risen in California, but needing to pay for more treatment to get more embryos on top of that simply meant it wasn't feasible to carry on. And that was aside from factoring in how physically broken I was and how mentally broken we both were.

This was it. The final whistle.

I don't remember much of what happened in the weeks after we decided to stop. Everyone who's ever

7. The club

been through IVF will know that deciding when to stop is a very individual process. In our case, we really had pushed every possibility to its limits and, although I desperately wanted to carry on, I knew there was no extra time to play. No other options left.

For six years, I'd been focused on how we would succeed. Or success as I saw it, anyway. Failure to deliver a family for us was just not a possibility I had been prepared to accept. But now I had to. And with that failure came an overwhelming guilt at not being able to give Lee the baby he wanted. In an angry rant, I would often tell him to go and find another woman who could have babies without this strife, and he would always assure me that his love was unconditional. Nevertheless, it was going to be another immense challenge to overcome those feelings of culpability.

In the weeks that followed, one day we were at home and we were both feeling really low. The sun was out and we were enjoying the garden. For some reason we just decided to crack open some bottles of lager left over from a gathering of friends at some point. I'm not sure why, because we would rarely drink at home. Of course, I'd spent years limiting my alcohol intake to try to control every parameter that might help me fall pregnant, and Lee almost never drinks at home either. But we had a drink, we had the beach towels laid out on the grass and we lay down, stroked our three doggies (affectionately known as our fur babies), and talked.

We talked about a reimagining of what success looked like for us. We talked about accepting where we were and accepting that children just might not happen for us now. We talked about moving away, possibly abroad, and creating an adventure. Lee said words I will never forget because they meant so much to me, though he probably didn't realise it. He said, "We'll build a different life together." It felt in that sentence as if I might, after all, be able to live again. To live a life with Lee, without living with the guilt of stripping him of his dreams. Without feeling as if I would have to leave him so he could be with someone else who *could* give him children. They were simple words, but they gave us a ticket to a future together.

In the end, we did more than just chat, if you get my drift. And it felt like after years of striving, we might both have accepted together that we needed to turn a corner. It was a sad day. But it was a good day. And we felt close to each other.

We booked a holiday to Ibiza the following month to try to nurture ourselves a little bit and get back to something as a couple that was beyond tests, treatments and trauma. But letting go isn't easy, and prior to leaving I did start to allow myself to get sucked back in. I wanted to see what the state of my insides was now, because the embryos from the IVF rounds in France and London kept popping into my head. They were now sitting in a new freezer home at the clinic in Wales. It was as if they were sitting there with a big 'What if?' sign accompanying them. We knew the chances of me falling pregnant and staying pregnant were slim, but I *had* managed to *fall* pregnant before Christmas and I couldn't help wanting to know if maybe, just maybe, something had improved in there.

Having asked my clinic in Wales to take a look, they advised me when I visited that nothing much had

7. The club

changed with my lining, but if we were to proceed with using the frozen embryos at all, I would need to get a small polyp removed first. I knew getting drawn back in was no good for me or us, but those little frosties waiting in the freezer were tiny little pieces of us waiting to be grown into a baby. It was too much to resist, so I booked the little op for after our return from Ibiza.

Ibiza, thankfully, did its job. We trained every day, we sunbathed, we ate, we swam. And we danced the night away in the club where Wham's 'Club Tropicana' video was filmed. Yes, we were probably drowning our sorrows to a degree, but it was fantastically cathartic. Being silly. Being drunk together. After so many years of only being serious and sad.

The clinic called me when we were there to confirm what date I could go in for the procedure, as it had to be done at a certain point in my cycle. I explained that I didn't quite know where I would be in my cycle when I got back as I was just waiting for my period to start. I assumed that the travelling and the training had thrown things off a bit.

The woman on the phone explained to me that we couldn't go ahead with the operation until I had my period and we knew my dates. I was gutted as I just wanted to get it done. Another barrier, another delay. In the end, we decided to put it all to one side until we got home and knew for certain where we were with the dates.

When we did get home, I needed to tell the clinic either way whether I was able to go in for this op. They said if my period was late, I needed to do a pregnancy test. At which I rolled my eyes, fairly frustrated, and said there was no chance that I could be pregnant. But they said if my period was late then they would not do the op until I had tested.

Well, I did the test. And we waited.

There were two very clear lines. And two very clear lines meant pregnant.

Even more incredibly, this had happened again with no treatment. This time we were not even in the run-up to a treatment cycle of any kind. Not a fertility drug in sight. After all science had told us, we seemed to be defying it.

We were dizzy with the swirl of hope versus reality. Petrified and excited in equal measure. A deep-seated fear of another failure forcing us to suppress the true joy with which we wanted to explode.

Unbelievably, six months on from a devastating miscarriage, it was here we go again. We were back in the game. We were in the club.

CHAPTER 8

Pip

(Please be aware that this chapter focuses on pregnancy and childbirth, and may be difficult to read if you are at a sensitive point on your fertility journey.)

WAITING. ALWAYS PAINFULLY waiting for something. With any optimism constantly at odds with the knowledge of what could go wrong. That's infertility. Especially long-term infertility, as you might now be realising. Even when there is a breakthrough – a major, major breakthrough like falling pregnant – joy has to be disabled, because the emotional risk is too high. Resist joy. Be numb.

It shouldn't be this way. We were pregnant again. It was the dream, after all, but all we did when we had that positive test was move from a lane of despair to a lane of anxiety. At this point of pregnancy, the majority of people would simply assume a nine-month journey to a baby ahead of them. For a couple like us, with a background of huge struggles and baby loss, it had to be a matter of taking it one day at a time.

But there was something I was quietly clinging on to – something which did seem too much of a coincidence. A month or so before I had this positive test, I'd taken a drug called doxycycline. It's a simple antibiotic – the type you might get prescribed for a chest infection, or the like. I wasn't prescribed it for chest infection, though.

In parallel to following the surrogacy path, over the previous year or so I had also remained in constant contact with my consultant in Wales, Amanda, who you'll remember had been with us at some of the lowest points. She said she would look for and flag up any new options for me. She told me about an NHS research trial that was happening in Coventry, which might be relevant to my particular diagnosis. I had committed myself to regular trips to Coventry and the joys of a doctor taking samples of my womb lining and testing them. I think I gave three samples (via quite a painful process which didn't grant you any anaesthetic and involved sucking a tiny piece of your womb lining away with a small implement of torture). The samples were tested and the results had revealed a couple of things.

As it turns out, my womb *didn't* have an excess of natural killer cells, which I had previously been told by the London clinic were in my blood, and which led me to try blood infusions to try to suppress or reduce them. It seemed when the test was more specifically done on a womb sample, rather than on a patient's blood, the result was more precise. And the killer cells weren't in my womb.

What the results did show, though, was that I had chronic inflammation or endometritis (not to be confused with endometriosis). In women it can be common and may not cause any issues, but if it does, it is relatively simple to treat.

It was this result that prompted those running the trial to prescribe me the antibiotic. I had tried it a couple of times up to this point – just to keep my options open, but never expecting anything. Well, guess what? A pattern

8. Pip

was developing. The last time I'd taken it was a little before our first trip to the US, when we'd found out we were pregnant. And the second time was prior to our IVF round in America. I'd decided to cover all bases prior to the treatment.

Now here we were, a month or so from that second US trip, and we had another positive pregnancy test. I felt something must be going on with how my lining was responding to the doxycycline. The ongoing trial hadn't yet proved if the drug worked – and I certainly don't know if there's any evidence that the effects of it remain helpful to your lining in the following months. But I felt as if was a connection. Perhaps last time when our tiny baby hadn't survived, the lining had been better, but the embryo was not of good quality. What we needed this time was for the lining to be better and the embryo to be of better quality too. The probabilities were low with my age and my history, but maybe – just maybe – this was it!

The first thing I did was get in touch with Amanda to see if I could go in for some extra scans. Ordinarily you don't get a scan until 12 weeks, but having lost a baby a couple of weeks earlier than that, I wanted to be reassured as much as I could. She said we could go for extra scans – once a week if we needed to – but would have to wait another month for the first scan, because until then it wouldn't be possible to see anything that resembled the beginnings of a baby, and even then we might not hear a heartbeat until a little further along.

Another wait. I remember life carried on as normal, but I wasn't wholly there. I had filming to do, voiceovers to complete, and I hosted a special live outside broadcast to celebrate the 70th anniversary of the NHS. Outside of work, we went to see Ed Sheeran and had a trip to Wimbledon. It was as if we were travelling through time but were existing in a different zone to everyone else around us. I wasn't completely present for anything during those first weeks, in particular. All I could think about was the little being that was (or wasn't) inside of me and whether I was capable of sustaining its life.

We went for a scan every Saturday for three weeks. On 21 July 2018, the consultant found a heartbeat and I cried my eyes out upon hearing it. I'd never thought I'd hear my baby's heartbeat. If we got no further, I had this to hold on to. It seemed unreal.

Sometimes we let ourselves believe. Just between the two of us. And I remember staying at my mum's for an ITV network news shift and looking at the old-school baby naming book which my own parents had used to name me and my sister. I loved that book. In the back, in my dad's handwriting, was their shortlist when my sister and I had been about to arrive. From that list, I knew I was almost a Zoe or a Marina! And if I'd been a boy, I would have been Andrew. Underneath that list, in my own childhood handwriting, was a list of what I might want to call my hamster too. Poppy or Penny were top contenders, though she actually ended up being a Dolly! But, in 2018, some of those names I fancied better for a human, truth be told. It was a lovely reminder of how times change and trends evolve.

Anyway, I found this little piece of my family story wonderful. I sat in bed looking through the book that night and sent a photo of it to Lee, daring to suggest some names I'd found. Whatever the future held, I suppose we both wanted in some way to enjoy the pregnancy like

8. Pip

any other couple might, even if it would make it harder later on. But we never decided on anything at this point. I think the fear of the jinx was too much. So, for the time being, we would call the baby Pip instead, because on a pregnancy monitoring app at some point it had compared the size of the foetus to that of an apple pip!

On 10 August, we had our 12-week scan. The all-important three months. Another point we had never reached. All looked well. Still we barely told anyone except close family and friends.

A few days later we chose to have extra tests early on to detect any abnormalities with the pregnancy. To be honest, I don't know what we expected to do with the results, but at that point in time we wanted to check everything we could. The test would also tell us the gender.

I remember telling my mum the results when she was on the train heading to see us in Wales. She already had two grandsons, who were at that point 10 and 14. Well, my mum won't mind me saying that she's not one to show emotion. I suppose she's of the wartime generation (born at the very end of the Second World War), where wearing your heart on your sleeve just wasn't done. So I was so touched when I told her on the phone that she was going to have a granddaughter and she was very emotional, immediately turning to the stranger who was sitting next to her to tell her.

It seemed like all was going to plan. However, I still didn't want to tell anyone at work. It was just too much to tell more people and feel that vulnerability if things should go wrong. In the next few weeks we did have a small scare. I went to the toilet at work and there was blood. Not much, but we'd been here before and I wasn't prepared to risk waiting. Fortunately, our clinic fitted me in almost immediately for a reassurance scan. There she was. Our baby. Heart still beating. Still growing.

At 15 weeks I did tell work, mostly because it was getting nearer to the point where I would be legally obliged to. Plus I felt as if I was beginning to look more than just a little bloated, so the more astute would probably soon be asking themselves the question anyway.

Then the 16-week scan passed, and the 20-week scan. As far as I recall, that's when they check all the limbs and organs are developing as they should be. I remember seeing her little feet kicking and her little hands reaching out. They gave me some scan photos I will cherish forever. I should at this point have felt a little more at ease. But, for me, I think 24 weeks was probably my threshold, because I knew at that point, had she needed to be delivered, she would have had a chance at surviving.

Until then I was paranoid. We had a 40th birthday trip planned for me in October to Formentera, a tiny island off Ibiza, but I was thinking of cancelling it at the last minute, afraid to travel given the miscarriage after travelling back from the US. But I thought about it over and over and tried to be realistic. The medics considered it safe in this trimester of pregnancy and those were the objective, rational voices I should listen to. Looking back on it now, I'm surprised I was brave enough to go, but I'm really glad we did. Sun, sea and sand probably did Pip the world of good – a lot more good than me sitting worrying at home. It goes without saying I had a very sober 40th! But for the best reason I could ever have wished for.

8. Pip

Without question, we cherished every moment of that pregnancy, from having a 3D scan so we could see the shape of her little face to organising a recording of her heartbeat to store inside a teddy bear. Whatever happened, we would have these things to keep.

Midwife appointments came and went with a lovely lady called Louise, who put up with my endless paranoia and was always reassuring.

Eventually 24 weeks came and I felt able to breathe just a little more easily. By December I felt confident enough to go to order cots, pram systems and all the baby paraphernalia, although I still refused to let the shop deliver any of it until a few weeks before my due date. The fear was still very real.

Similarly, one of my colleagues offered to organise a baby shower for me, but I just couldn't bring myself to do it. Just in case. It felt like I could jinx something if I was too confident. It sounds ridiculous, but anyone who has been on the fertility rollercoaster or lost babies will know that paranoia.

By January, about seven weeks before Pip's due date, I was brave enough to commission a cartoon for the nursery. It features me with Lee – I'm clutching a bunch of news scripts and he has his foot on a rugby ball. In his arm he's cradling an upside-down hard hat, in which sits little Pip. The hard hat was a subtle nod to Lee's new business development career in the construction industry, but also a metaphor for building our future and the rest of our family. Our family prior to Pip's arrival, the three dogs (yes, we had three now!), are at our feet.

This I intended to hang alongside the piece of wooden wall art we had bought in San Jose, on that impromptu road trip when we had fallen pregnant in America. The wall art said, 'Grateful. Thankful. Blessed.' It had been brought back to Wales in our suitcase, and then hidden away in the garage, associated with difficult memories. But I knew I would hang it up if Pip came to be with us, in that little nursery we had so longed to fill. One part of me hated the sentiment of being 'blessed' because we had managed to have a baby, because I felt it implied that those who might *not* be so fortunate somehow weren't worthy enough to be 'blessed' and granted their dream. But another part of me liked the fact that it reminded me of where and why we'd bought it. It symbolised all that we'd been through and was a tribute to the babies that were gone, but certainly not forgotten.

All in all, I was slowly gaining confidence in this pregnancy and suppressing my paranoia. I also turned to work as a coping strategy. Perhaps not the healthiest option as I should ideally have been winding down, but I did feel worried about leaving my job behind after 11 years at the helm, presenting the news. I'm not sure it matters what you do: it is a weird transition to go on maternity leave and watch someone else do your job. For me, it somehow helped to prepare myself by throwing myself into producing a series of exclusive reports on subjects close to my heart, like rising sepsis deaths – to raise awareness in my dad's name – and mental health provision. I remember filming with a police patrol late into the night just a month or so before my due date. I guess I was somehow trying to prove my worth before I left, which in hindsight was uncalled for. Ladies, I implore you: don't feel this way! That job is yours and will be there when you return.

8. Pip

My last day in work finally came around and I was sent off with a huge cheer as I left the studio for the last time – for the time being. There were some lovely parting gifts and, coincidentally, I started my maternity leave on the same day that my best friend Carl – who had helped me through so much in the previous few years and come to appointments as moral support when Lee was bound to rugby fixtures – left to start another job. It felt quite appropriate that we were moving on to a new era in both our lives together.

In the last few weeks, I seemed to absolutely balloon. My abdominal area, of course, but also my hands, face and ankles just seemed to start getting puffier and puffier. Sleeping, eating... everything was a struggle. The symptoms of late pregnancy were accelerating.

It was, fittingly, on Valentine's Day – 14 February 2019 – that we knew it really wouldn't be long before we would meet the much-longed-for love of our lives. Having been for lunch with some friends, I remember telling them how my hands and feet seemed to be ever-expanding and that I felt like I was auditioning to be the Michelin Man's understudy. It seemed something different was happening that hadn't occurred before in my pregnancy. Pip wasn't due for another 10 days, though, so I was relatively dismissive of it all. Plus, everyone kept telling me first babies arrive late. However, let me think: when had our fertility story ever stuck to the script?

Sure enough, Pip continued to defy the norm. That night I was in bed and felt the need to wee urgently. Just as I got close to the toilet, whoosh! There was water everywhere. When they say your waters break, they really do. It was a flood.

I shouted for Lee, to tell him what had happened, and it seemed to take an incredible number of calls to wake him from his slumber. At least one of us was getting a good night's rest! Eventually he realised what was happening. We gathered our thoughts, called the hospital and set off to the maternity ward – by now in the early hours of 15 February. This I think Lee was secretly chuffed about, as 15 was his full back shirt number and he'd always considered 15 to be particularly good luck. It also crossed my mind that a Valentine's birthday probably wouldn't have been much fun when little Miss Byrne was trying to go for a birthday dinner and everything was booked up or triple the price!

It did look and feel to me as if we were all set for labour, but actually when we arrived at the hospital, they did some monitoring and checking and then sent us home. I wasn't expecting this. To be sent away from the reassurance of experts was not good for the fragility of my nerves. But away we went, to wait for the contractions to start coming far more closely together.

What I did vaguely know, though, was that it was better to give birth sooner rather than later once your waters had broken, because of the risk of infection to the baby. So I started doing everything I could to encourage Pip out. We went for a really long walk along the Porthcawl coastal path, we ate lots of curry (not sure if that's a myth or not!) and I was bouncing gently on my big exercise ball. Mid-morning it felt like the contractions were getting more painful and closer together, so we went back in around lunchtime.

I was put on a machine to monitor Pip's heartbeat and taken straight into a labour room. There seemed to

8. Pip

be some concerns that they wanted to keep an eye on, so I remained on the machine. My contractions were now much closer together and much more painful. I was on gas and air and motivating myself with the soundtrack to *The Greatest Showman*. Lee was here, there and everywhere. I don't think he knew what to do with himself. He'd be up and down, in and out, grabbing coffee after coffee. There was a facial mist I'd brought with me and I remember asking him to spray me to cool me down and he just kept spraying me really close up over and over until I was dripping! I didn't have the heart to tell him it was a little full on. We were both on edge and jumpy, after all.

Time ticked on, as did the labour, but I wasn't dilating very much, which didn't seem to make sense to me – or to anyone else. This went on for hours. It was now early evening and despite contraction after contraction, when they measured me, things hadn't really progressed a lot.

Meanwhile, the baby's heartbeat was also not measuring exactly as it should either.

At this stage I don't think they fully explained the problem to me, but I knew there *was* a problem. What I do remember is that suddenly a lot started happening very quickly. Lots of people were suddenly in the room and I was told I was having an epidural with a view to preparing for an emergency Caesarean section. This meant I would be numbed from the waist down to allow for the serious abdominal surgery to take place. Or to put it more flippantly, Pip had to come out through the sunroof.

Before I knew it, I was being moved to theatre. What we didn't know then but soon found out was that the umbilical cord had wrapped around her neck three times, which meant she was head first and trying to push down to the exit, but the cord was so short, she kept getting pulled back up again, like on a bungy. Which in turn meant I wasn't dilating and she could be struggling to breathe. The medics must have had a pretty good idea of this, as they decided to move so quickly to the op. But, thankfully, we were ignorant and therefore felt relatively calm and able to put our trust in the professionals.

I'd never experienced an anaesthetic like this, nor any major surgery. It was very strange to be able to feel lots of pulling and pushing going on inside my tummy area, but be unable to feel any pain. Lee and I had no choice but to believe what was happening behind that green screen was going to plan and Pip was safely on her way to us. We held each other's hands, urging the moment to come when we could hold on to hers.

Eventually it did. At 8.27 p.m. on 15 February, our tiny, precious and perfect miracle baby was brought into the world.

We called her Jemima Hazel Rhona Byrne. Jemima in Hebrew means 'dove'. A symbol of peace, freedom and hope.

Hazel was in memory of Lee's aunt who had passed away too soon from cancer and Rhona in memory of my nana, who we lost when I was just 11.

Grateful. Thankful. Blessed.

And painfully aware that not everyone experiences such a joyous end to their story.

Epilogue

(A letter from me to Jemima, to explain what happened next)

Dearest Jemima,

As I write this, you may or may not be starting to realise how special you are.

Maybe you know all too well. I hope so. But not in a way that ruins you!

Although I admit that will be hard. How can we not overprotect you, over-provide for you, over-love you, over-compliment you? After all, you silenced the science. You proved that theories are there to be rewritten. You are a medical marvel.

I tell you all the time that you're our little miracle. I remember once messages got confused. I'd also been trying to explain your heritage. That Mummy's family were English and Daddy's Welsh. I said one day, "Remember you're our little miracle," and you turned around, all confused, and said, "No, I'm not, I'm half English." That did make us chuckle. And then you started chuckling, though you'd no idea why. Then that made us chuckle more. That giggle. That infectious happiness. That joy.

We had many years of medical help to try to have you. Life is complex and it turns out some people find it easier to create babies and grow them than others. In our case, this took a particularly long while. And, in the end, despite all the medical help we tried, you decided of your own accord when the time was right to come along – and you were more than worth the wait! The magic happened and you grew and grew from a tiny Pip to a wonderful little baby – and, at the time of writing, a 5-year-old little girl. Incredible, inquisitive and unstoppable.

You've given us everything we ever dreamed of and more. And with that, you also inspired us. If *you* happened this once, maybe another you could happen.

I think something shifted in me after we had you. Emotionally, of course it did. I was a mother, after all. But also physically. It felt as if, well, my body really did know how to create a baby, grow a baby and birth one. So I wanted you to know that when we felt ready, we decided to try to see if there was any chance we could gift you a baby brother or sister.

And, sweetheart, it almost happened. We returned to science to help us a little as we already had little embryos – the very beginnings of a baby – stored in a freezer from when we'd been trying to have you. Through one part of a clever process called IVF, we did fall pregnant again. We really thought this was it. We had the belief this time. It wasn't like before. We had a renewed confidence that it could be.

I was not only convinced it would all be OK again, but I was also sure it was a boy and even had a name ready – I'll tell you one day. I wanted to keep mentally strong and so I was keeping physically strong. I was walking a lot with you, Daddy and our fur babies. Every walk I did, I felt as if I was walking to your brother.

We were once again going for regular check-ups to make sure he was on track. And he seemed to be. We were getting closer and closer to that 12-week mark. But, for

Epilogue

reasons we will never know, he couldn't make it through. Maybe my womb – where babies grow – couldn't give him what he needed. Maybe my age played a part. We'll never know. But we had to say goodbye.

What seemed like weeks later, we fell pregnant once again. My body wanted this. *We* wanted this. For us, for you. This time it was a fainter line on the test, a fainter sign that there was a tiny baby in my tummy, but nonetheless we still thought, 'Maybe'. The line soon faded as we retested.

This happened twice. The briefest of hellos and the quickest of goodbyes.

And whilst I will always be so proud of what Daddy and I did – and of course what you did – to create our little family, I will always be sad in my soul that I couldn't give you a baby brother or sister. I know you would have been the best of older sisters. I see you with your younger cousin and how you are a natural mother hen. Or maybe rather a Jemima puddle duck – you lead and the little ones follow. The same with our dogs – how much you care, how much love you have to give to them. I see you playing with your dolls in the same tender way.

You have asked me every so often why you don't have a brother or a sister, which breaks my heart. Or should I say, 'scrumples my heart' – a gorgeous phrase you came home with one day from school. I've tried to explain that it took a long time for us to make you. I remember I was driving and you were sitting in the back of the car thinking about all this. You were asking me questions about things that had happened in the past. Maybe a holiday we'd talked about going on before you existed in the world. I could almost hear your small but inquisitive brain working. You were trying to work out why you weren't around when certain things had happened. After a few minutes you said to me, "So if I wasn't there then, did God just take a really long time to make me?"

I said, "That's pretty much it, Jemima."

So please know: we tried to add another one to our team. So you had a crew. For when times get tough. And for when we might not be around. But eventually our luck, and our time, ran out.

But as time moves on, it only means we savour every moment with you more. Knowing that already we have now been blessed with several fabulous years of Jemima. Some people will call you an only child, but I call you my one and only. A wonderful whirlwind who has changed *our* world – and I've no doubt will change *the* world.

Making Babies

podcast stories

In the following section, the information given relates to the time of recording (see panel at start of each story for date).

CLARE NASIR

On fibroids and fertility

> **Clare Nasir** is a weather presenter for Channel 5 and an author. For decades, she lived with the pain of large fibroids, which hindered her fertility. Her journey – with her husband, BBC Radio 6 Music DJ Chris Hawkins – was far from easy. Here she shares those experiences and sheds light on the little-talked-about condition of fibroids and the far-reaching and complex effects they can have, both physically and emotionally. Clare and Chris have a daughter called Sienna.
>
> 🎧 *Podcast released on 25 October 2021.*

Our daughter is just the best thing in our lives and we call her our miracle baby. She's 11 now and she's just so perfect and beautiful and wise – cooler than I'll ever be. Everything about her is just perfect. There's lots of unknowns going out there into the big bad world and making that transition to high school, but she's embraced it all. She's got some of my temperament and some of Chris' as well – overall she's just incredible. I think there's a lot of pressure when you have one child, making up for all the other siblings who aren't with us, but she is doing a good job being the only one.

I knew I had problems before I met Chris, my husband. I remember going to see my grandma, who was a real y and had been through the war and everything – she was quite hard really, but an amazing woman. I'd just been diagnosed with fibroids and I remember telling her that I had acute fibroids and it was just like the blood drained from her face. Back in her day when you had fibroids, you had a hysterectomy – end of. And this is her granddaughter, her oldest granddaughter, who was in her early thirties then. She had three kids herself and thought I wasn't going to be blessed with children. Thankfully, things are different now in the twenty-first century, and I've had a number of procedures which helped me.

It was hell, though, it really was. Fibroids are just vile. You feel like there's an alien inside you just sucking the life out of you. I think I waited too long to have a diagnosis and it was probably six years of my life where I was just rolling from exhaustion to the next procedure, and at the back of my mind, I didn't think I could have children. After I met Chris, I said to him that I probably wouldn't ever be able to have kids but he still proposed – so there you go.

When I went to the doctor's, I just felt like I had constipation and a solid stomach. I didn't know what fibroids were at that stage, but it ended up pretty much ruining my early thirties really, particularly with the pain and blood loss. I was diagnosed eventually with fibroids, which are benign tumours. They live in your womb and most of the time they're not cancerous or nasty, but they live off blood so they sort of just really want to suck that blood out of you. The largest one, at its biggest, was about the size of a rugby ball. So I looked around four to five months pregnant before I had my first procedure.

I opted for a uterine embolization, which is a keyhole surgery, which severs all the ties with the surrounding blood vessels and slowly the beast dies inside you, but it dies over six months to a year and the cramping involved during that time, as it's sort of withering and lashing out for more blood, is really painful and quite debilitating.

I met Chris around this time and as soon as we were married, he wanted to support me in sorting it all out, because the symptoms were still there. So I went on to the next level of operation, which was a myomectomy. It's almost like having a caesarean but they're taking out the tumour, and in fact my gynaecologist at the time said it was good that I'd had the embolization first because it had shrunk from a size of a rugby ball to the size of a grapefruit, so it was easier to get out.

Before the operation, they took my blood and they said, "You're highly anaemic." I didn't realise, but I remember not being able to get up the stairs. So they gave me a blood transfusion and took me into the theatre. I remember I ended up being in there a lot longer than I should have been and Chris was scared – I think it took its toll, with the worry and trying to keep both our families informed. I think in that moment reality kicked in and he just decided that we should try for children. Whereas me, I just wanted to skip down the road for a few years and just have a bit of fun now that procedure was out of the way!

When I was ready, we paid to see a really respected gynaecologist in Harley Street. We were conscious of my age and he'd done one of my procedures. He said my womb was a battlefield. So I had another procedure to tidy up my womb: a laparoscopy, another procedure with general anaesthetic. I'd now had three proper procedures to really get myself back on track.

We tried to conceive naturally for a few years before moving on to IVF, but nothing happened and it was quite disheartening. Chris comes from a family of three and I had more siblings than that and it's amazing being part of a massive family, I absolutely love it. I'm really proud to have all my brothers around me at any point and so I wanted a big family. Your thirties is when you're meant to have children and once you get into your forties, every year, you know you're losing another year and I was sick of the pressure. All my brothers and Chris' sisters were having kids, and all my friends were.

I remember going through the first few failures of IVF and Kate Garraway coming into work and saying, "I'm pregnant." Kate is my best friend and we shared a dressing room together at GMTV, and I was so happy for her and so sad for me. Chris also kept saying, "I see pregnant women everywhere, everyone's pregnant. How does this happen? I never saw pregnant women in my twenties!" It becomes all-consuming, affecting everything. I think it does. I remember, I think after my first failure or maybe my second, we were on the Southbank in London and having drinks with some friends, and I felt a bit numb really, but Chris was sad. I remember a lovely friend of mine – Carla Romano, who was the LA Correspondent – noticing Chris. She gave him the biggest bear hug and you could see him just thinking, 'Someone understands.' I don't think we were really communicating on that level whilst we were on the treadmill and I think Chris probably felt it more than I did because it was more out of his control.

It also affected me professionally. With my fibroids, it was hard because I looked so pregnant towards the end before I had my operations, and people were emailing in and just saying, "Why is Clare Nasir not telling anyone she's pregnant?" You also want to look good on TV and people called me 'chunky Nasir' for a while. I was on a cruise just before my first operation and there was one of these scavenger hunts and one of the things the kids had to do was to find a pregnant lady. I had so many kids running up to me and saying, "Can you sign my form?" But I wasn't pregnant.

My heart goes out to anyone who's going through the same thing with fibroids because I think they're really nasty. I had a good set of really strong women around me at work, which helped. I had Fiona Phillips, Penny Smith, Kate Garraway and Lorraine Kelly fighting my corner, so when it came to the IVF, I was very lucky in that respect. Even so, I still had to do my job and three days out of the five I was travelling around the country broadcasting to north, south, east and west, and I was taking all my IVF equipment with me. I had my injections and so on, and was somehow trying to fit in the appointments at the hospital. And obviously there was disappointment afterwards, and that happened a number of times. I think you do end up saying to yourself, "I'm just going to be focused. There is a happy end point to this and I'm a very positive person and it will eventually happen for me." Though obviously that positivity wanes when you get your fourth negative pregnancy test.

I think it's also important to say that fibroids can come back. It can be down to diet, or maybe down to stress. Tumours manifest for so many different reasons.

It's like infertility. Who knows what it comes down to? It's just tragically the worst luck, really. So that was my thirties, pretty much. Then – bang! – straight into fertility treatment. I think that time in my life was hard overall. I was always involved in something gynaecological.

Eventually, we did have a positive result. But the drama wasn't over for me when I got pregnant. Those first few weeks were quite tentative and even a few months were quite bad. Sienna ended up being premature. She really, really was my miracle. I started haemorrhaging at 9 weeks and went into the early clinics to get reassurance, so I think she was the most photographed baby ever. We found a heartbeat at about 9 or 10 weeks, which was still strong even though I was bleeding. My waters then broke at 21 weeks, though, so I rushed to hospital, where they thought I would either miscarry or give birth at any point.

I remember them taking me into a ward – an isolated ward, because of infection – and I said, "I'm keeping this baby inside me." I was then really determined that I was going to get through this and keep her inside as long as I could. When she was 21 weeks, she was a pound. She was like a little bag of sugar and then they said, "We just want two bags of sugar" – that's all we wanted.

I discharged myself from the hospital because I was going mad. I begged GMTV to take me back to work but they said no. I was supposed to avoid people because of the risk of infection to the baby, but found myself occasionally just going, "I'm going to sit in the pub for half an hour with a book and just have a bit of normal life during the middle part of the day when there's no-one around," because I just needed a little bit of normality.

It wasn't a happy pregnancy, but the nearer I got to 30 weeks, the greater the chance that everything was going to be OK.

She came at 30 weeks, maybe 30 and a half. One morning, Chris was going to work at 3 o'clock (he presents the early-morning slot on 6 Music) and I was getting all these stomach pains. He left and I just called a cab and took myself off to the same amazing hospital which had saved Sienna's life so far. I just knew it would be OK at this stage. I remember texting Chris, who was on air at the time, saying, "I'm going into the theatre soon, so you better run." The BBC studios are two blocks away and he finished on air at 7.30 a.m. and literally ran to the hospital, where I was all gowned up, ready to go in. Five epidurals later, because they didn't work, a little, little tiny baby came out. She was a little girl. She was three and a half pounds and she was in intensive care within moments and she was there for quite a while. She had to have a lot of physio at first, because there'd been no fluid around her for nine weeks.

We were back and forth to the hospital for a long while. Chris got a cab into work every morning at 3.30 so I'd jump in with him and sit by her bed and wait, wait for that moment when she could be released. And there were a couple of times where the blue lights went off, and the doctors just pushed me out of the room and everyone came and descended on her to save her. She was in a ward with six other babies and I'm still in contact with some of those mums now. In fact, one of the mums was Martha Wainwright, the singer. Martha used to sing to her little boy whilst we were all there. So there was a lot of emotion in that neonatal ward. It's a place of hope and it's a place where miracles happen, but those corridors can be very dark.

Sienna came out of hospital just before Christmas. It started snowing and we put her in a little snowsuit.

I begged to go back to work really early after Sienna was born, because I needed to. In fact about two weeks after Sienna came home, I called them and asked, "Can I come in with the baby?" There's a photo with Emma Crosby, Andrew Castle and Kate Garraway. We were sitting on the GMTV sofa with the Christmas tree still up and Andrew is holding her in one hand. She was so tiny – she was five and a half pounds by then, so that was a lovely moment. Sienna has seen that on YouTube quite a lot.

As time went on, we did at some point decide to use the frozen embryos we had too, but they failed. I had to close the door on it. It was just one of those things where you think, 'Actually, we've got our miracle baby, and she's amazing.' We went down the adoption route for a while as well, because we did want other children, but after the first stage of going through that and seeing the social workers, we felt that we weren't aligned in what we wanted and so we closed that door as well. Since then it's just been us three, living a brilliant life.

I've really embraced life since Sienna. Even just the other day, Chris thought it was just me and him in the garden sipping wine, but I'd invited the whole street round. I live for the day. I love being here and now and just marvelling at even the smallest thing. I think it was maybe what I needed to go through to whip me into shape so I had a good attitude to life, because prior to that I always felt there was something better around the corner – I was in that quagmire of despair when I just wanted things to be normal again. I wanted to be able to just sit down and not have to think about all the hospital stuff.

We've moved north now and I've met some amazing people up here. A network of mums is really important in the early stages, particularly when you've been through so much trauma over so many years. You've been in a cave and that cave has been quite damp and dark and quite cold in places, and you come out into the shiny light and it blinds you a little bit. But I can now focus on the positive.

GEOFF NORCOTT

On stillbirth and men's mental health

> **Geoff Norcott** is a well-known British comedian. Although his job on stage is to make people laugh, *off* the stage he and his wife Emma have experienced huge sadness through the trauma of losing a baby. He is now a dedicated supporter of the stillbirth and neonatal death charity SANDS, and a pioneer for men's mental health. To help raise awareness, he agreed to share the story of their daughter, Connie. They went on to have a son called Sebastian.
>
> 🎧 Podcast released on 19 April 2022.

I have sat down many times to write articles about losing our daughter, Connie. It is a topic so under-discussed. Eventually I wrote an article for SANDS, and it was constructive but difficult for me.

As part of the grieving process, it's interesting in terms of, 'Where am I this week?' It's so hard to work out what your subconscious is doing. But there are certain little psychological pointers that tell me that that's what I'm upset about, and one of them is that I just don't feel that anything I've ever done is good or anything's going well – that I've sort of failed. Things that I thought were successes, I suddenly think were failures. I think that's part of the process of beating yourself up – like you're culpable, like you did something wrong.

My wife Emma is quite a private person so she's found it really difficult, and she found it harder than she thought she would when the SANDS article went a bit more viral than anyone expected. She found it hard that our neighbours then knew details about our life, and she was torn between being very sad yet also delighted for me, because she knew that it was something that I needed to do.

I don't regret it, as there was such a skimpy amount of discourse in this area and I was looking to find out what that weird feeling is, that thing you can't explain: 'Am I mad?', 'Is it just me?' A lot of counselling therapy is all about that and the more dramatic the circumstances and more specific the feeling, the more that you need counselling. So, I knew that there was something I could offer by speaking out and I think it's been a positive thing. We realise, I think, that Connie's memory is more of a thing now. People mention her name to me and the correspondence was quite a lot, really.

I suppose her name being mentioned is really nice, but it can be jarring, because it's that thing that's made real by being reflected back to you. We always discussed her with friends and family and with each other, we weren't one of those couples that buried it deep down. But it's a double-edged sword because if you're having a certain kind of day and then you hear that name or you see it written down, it's hard.

Men process grief in a different way, I think, too. I think there's a problem that counselling and therapy is often a bit female-led in terms of language. I don't necessarily want to bring class into it, but I think for working class blokes it's especially true. I remember going to see a counsellor and she said to me, "Oh, it's okay to be weak." I didn't want to talk about weakness. And then she would say to me, "What you're talking about is brave." And I thought, 'It's not brave either.' I think there's a sort of functional view that men have of these things. And if you can put it to men in a functional way, that can do a lot of the work. I mean, when I speak to my pals about counselling or therapy, I just talk about it like a pit stop – like maintenance.

You can't deny that the brain is the most finely tuned thing that we know of on planet Earth. It's just so complex and magical and weird. So the idea that you would need to do things to have running repairs on that often works, in terms of speaking to blokes. The other thing is that a lot of blokes just simply don't think that it works. And one of the things that I always tell them is about the amount of money that the US military invests in talking therapies, because a lot of blokes will just go, "They've got the best army. If they're doing something, then there must be some merit in it." It's these little weird ways that you can get into the conversation.

One of my friends said to me when I did eventually go for counselling, "The more you put in, the more you get out." You have to somehow challenge the view that it's manly to not talk. That's the hardest thing, because if the consequence of not talking is that you engage in destructive behaviours, then you know you end up not taking care of your responsibilities.

When we were told we had lost Connie, I think the process was quite clinical. Then having to go home for two days, knowing that the labour was still going to happen, was tough. No-one spoke to us or visited us at that time, or offered support. That period of time, it's every bit as sad and traumatic as people would think. There were social workers up to a point. They looked in on us and that was a weird experience in itself, to have people monitoring you. In terms of friends, it was hard because the focus is rightly centred on the woman. I think that as a bloke, you do have someone to care for – you have your wife, who will come back from the hospital feeling fairly broken, emotionally and physically, and who needs your constant care and attention. You can throw yourself into that quite willingly in a lot of ways, because the feeling is so strong to try and look after them. It's very easy for people to always ask about your wife, but a few months in and then probably it's the right time for them to talk to you about it – but then they're all thinking, 'It was six months ago... it was a year ago...', so they might not bring it up. But for you, it's yesterday.

One thing I think you do have to do is to tell a lot of people. You sort of become a news reporter in your own life, taking solace in reporting to people what they need to know. I do think that sometimes that's a mistake blokes make: they think it's respectful to never talk about it. But that can lead to you just feeling like you're in a surreal vacuum where this life-changing event has happened and no one ever talks about it.

It can also be that, after a while, you notice that your wife is recovering a bit, and she's recovered her spirits a little bit, but you're going down. But you sort of think, 'I should probably just take this one on myself.' It's almost impossible that you're both going to want to talk about it at the same time. And there are not many griefs in life that are like that, that you share exactly with somebody.

The other really tough thing is that I see my son become more incredible and brilliant and fascinating and complex. By the time they get to five and a half, they're very distinctive personalities. And like so many things with stillbirth, you're projecting into a void. With other griefs, you have memories, you have things. In this, you don't really. So you have to go through the process of almost constructing a relationship to then grieve it.

There'll be times where there'll be girls of a certain age and I think of Connie. I also notice fathers with their daughters. I can remember there was a guy with his daughter, and he just went to the toilet with the baby bag and he obviously did what he needed to do and came out. He looked so competent and I was so jealous of him. When you think about being a father, there are certain instincts that you have that remain unfulfilled, such as the desire to protect. And I have that with my son, obviously, but with girls it's different. And the way that you decorate a room and the little dresses that you buy and all these little things you see around and about are delicate reminders of what you were expecting. It breaks you down into your constituent pieces, really.

The experience and the emotion has definitely affected my work.

What I kind of hoped after all this grief that I went through was that I'd never get nervous again – that I'd sort of think, 'There are bigger things in life.' It's just a comedy gig. But I also think I have a legacy of anxiety. I can get very low and very exhausted when I have to carry on working while these things are going on in my brain. So when you feel compromised when you go out on stage, it's not a good feeling. You know, you go out, you feel tired, you feel dizzy. There are a few hundred people there and you've got to be up there an hour, which can be pretty tough.

It's really hard because you sort of think, 'Am I a wiser person?' We lost Connie and my mum – and I think until your first parent goes or your first big grief, you just don't really believe you're gonna die or that stuff goes wrong. And then the moment that happens, you sort of feel the tectonic plates shift beneath you. That's another thing that I've spoken a lot about in terms of male mental health: the anxiety that comes from grief. A lot of people think, 'Oh, I'll just be sad sometimes', but it can be sadness, anger, and anxiety. I think culturally women will gather round one another in these situations, but blokes aren't as well versed in what's going on.

For me, the emotion definitely manifested as anxiety. I could cope with the depression, and I feel sad but that's quite a safe place to be. But sometimes in a weird way, once that shifts and you see the world more vividly and sharply, it can be a bit overwhelming. I felt like I was orbiting my own life for a while. I've had several spells where the anxiety has become unmanageable. That's usually also to do with exhaustion, illness and overwork. So, I've had several spells on anti-anxiety medication, which again, I didn't ever want to do. But I have responsibilities to my family. So, I have to be functional on a certain level and I can't completely concertina.

I had plenty of counselling. But one thing I've learned about counselling is that you have to know when to change counsellors, because sometimes you just have the same conversation. And there is a point with counsellors where you're just moaning – it's not constructive. But

I think talking therapies are something I believe in. It's almost like a form of alchemy where you can go through a conversation, then you just happen upon a thing, you go to say it, you choke up, and that's the best bit. And a lot of people fight that bit. It's like a form of magic to me. And then you can have some sessions where you don't get any of that, and I think I want a refund!

The other things that help are the ways we remember Connie. There's a place that we go that's a memorial place. And then obviously there's the places where her ashes are. And she's very much in the language of my son. He knows who she is. I was always unsure about that. It's very early in life to know, but equally for our sanity we needed to be able to mention her. I think that *is* constructive. We'll mark certain anniversaries and sometimes I'll see how Emma is feeling and I'll just say, "Get in the car – go, go see her." Every once in a while, you go and sit there and you feel something, or you are aware of how that experience shaped you for the better, or made you a better parent or more appreciative of things. But it's never an easy trip.

As a parent to Sebastian, I think it has probably made us a bit more risk-averse, but I think the main things are internal. It definitely made me savour being a parent more, but also sometimes it can be hard to let yourself enjoy the wondrous things. You feel bad because it's a different timeline from Connie and that can be hard to square. And sometimes there are points where he becomes so much more incredible. Every time you think that it couldn't be more magical, it is. He's a very magical little man. There's something very special about him and that has got us through a lot.

Making Babies podcast: Geoff Norcott

There's also survivor's guilt. One thing I've learnt, particularly through losing my best friend as well, is that it's a really strange thing. It's a very powerful emotion. Why am I still around and they're not? If you look at soldiers, they get it a lot. I remember I was watching the film *Dunkirk*, about who gets off the beach, who gets to live and who doesn't. And it absolutely crushed me. And I had some counselling after that and that turned out to be the thing I was carrying most in relation to him. Grief is so non-linear, so complicated, magical and dark. It's an absolute beast, but it does make me think that humans are fundamentally good because the way that we feel about losing people that we love, it's just so deep and constant.

I've certainly become a bit more empathetic. It was Connie's five-year anniversary in 2019 and my mum's tenth one. Something shifted in me a little bit, and I talk about it a fair bit in the book, but I came out the other side of that a bit less angry, perhaps. I still love debates, I still have my views and stuff, but I wasn't angry with anybody any more, I found.

Less anger but still a lot of anxiety. I just don't allow myself to enjoy the idea of the future. That's hard: to think ahead and think, 'It's gonna be good.'

If there is anyone who needs some help through the immediate aftermath of trauma right now, I would say to make life as easy for yourself as possible. Acknowledge the exhaustion you must be feeling. If you can't feel happy, or don't want to feel happy, be honest with yourself. You have to deal with that. 'But why, why don't I want to feel happier?' And the truth is probably, people will often feel that they don't deserve to be, or that they did something wrong and they're sort of putting themselves through a hard time as an act of contrition, or as a tribute to whoever they've lost. At least if you acknowledge – 'I'm being hard on myself' or 'I'm beating myself up', you might just ease off a little bit, even if it doesn't stop it completely. If you can just work out that you're punishing yourself, then that's the start of a new way of thinking about it.

Finally, I would just recommend people to go to the support charities, especially **SANDS**. The subject matter can be tricky, so they don't always get a lot of publicity.

RIA & FERN BURRAGE-MALE

On IVF and sperm donation for same-sex couples

> **Ria Burrage-Male** is a former International hockey player for Wales, and former CEO of Hockey Wales. She is married to former footballer, now coach, **Fern Burrage-Male**. As a same-sex couple, Ria and Fern spoke to me about the complexities of choosing a sperm donor, their rollercoaster with IVF and the pros and cons of either of them being able to carry the baby.
>
> 🎧 Podcast released on 14 February 2022.

Ria: Fern and I had been friends before we actually became a couple. I retired from international sports and realised there was a bit of a gap in my life, and I knew straight away that I wanted to start a family. I was on my own at the time and I just thought, 'I'm going to do it.' So I initially started the ball rolling and went through the NHS to start the process. Maybe that's my sports mentality. I knew that was the next step for me, so I didn't really give any thought to what it would actually be like being a single mum. I just knew I had a good network of people around me anyway.

Then I got together with Fern and she already knew what I was doing because we were friends, so it just really worked out well in that sense. I just continued with the NHS and we had a conversation, agreeing that we'd see what would happen and take it from there.

At that time I was unsuccessful. I had the egg extraction but unfortunately the embryos which were created hadn't developed and weren't strong enough, and the pregnancy failed. We chatted and thought, 'This is a sign, so let's try something different.' Our relationship had progressed and we decided that we would maybe carry for each other. So we contacted a local clinic and had an appointment with them, and we decided in the initial instance that Fern would carry my eggs. So that was the next step then on our IVF journey as a couple. All of that happened over two years, I'd say.

Fern: It was interesting because, as Ria said, I knew she was on this journey. I'd always wanted a family. I'd done the very, very initial exploration of it myself because I was completely naive about how it might work for me. I didn't want to stop what Ria was doing because I didn't know what our relationship looked like at the initial stages. But it wasn't until there were more appointments and I started to be more involved, and our relationship grew, that it became very much that we were *both* on this journey. Within the first 12 to 18 months, it turned into our journey together.

I think right from the start I'd say it's hard being the person looking on whilst your partner has treatment. We've had a number of attempts at IVF through both the NHS and privately and we've both been in both positions, because we've done Ria's eggs in Ria, we've done Ria's eggs in me, and now we've done my eggs in

Making Babies podcast: Ria & Fern Burrage-Male

Ria. So, fortunately, as the journey has progressed, we've both had the opportunity to be the person in it and also the person who has to hold the hand, almost, and it is incredibly difficult. I guess we're blessed in the way that we've both been in both positions. Some couples don't experience that. So we can really empathise with what they're going through and that really makes a difference. Being in a same-sex couple and the way we've done it has really helped us.

That's one side where we have more choices, but on the flip side, we have to buy some sperm! One evening we had to get the laptop out and a glass of wine and start searching for a donor. We were a bit giggly with it at the start. I imagine it's like a dating app. You do some filtering, such as ticking 'dark hair' as we both have dark hair. We knew we wanted someone fit and healthy. Then there's the more serious stuff. You get a full medical history, but you also get the full medical history of the parents and the grandparents and siblings, which is excellent, but you then start getting further details, such as did they wear glasses or have braces? And then the kind of sillier stuff: what food do they like? Who's their celebrity look-alike? And you start saying, "Oh, they like country music, so do we!" It's the smallest of things you might use to narrow down the search because they might all fit the bill, but something has to differentiate between them. And it doesn't really matter, but you've got five in front of you. How do you pick one over the other? Or they show you pictures. Do you want to see pictures?

Ria: I didn't want to. I blocked it out. It's a process. Also it's down to chromosome deficiencies and medical history, so if I had a condition that I don't know about and that donor had a condition and we matched, that creates a risk. As Fern said, ultimately the donor's health is the most important thing. But you can see things like handwriting, photos, baby photos of them – and I've blanked all that out now. I think you've still got a bit of a memory of it, but it's just science for me, which is how I deal with it.

Fern: I think I'm just not worried about it. I don't see the donor as a part of it – as involved in this. I have seen a baby photo from their original profile and it doesn't bother me. I know that we didn't order a UK donor and that was important to us. I didn't want to ever be thinking, "Did I just walk past him? Did I bump into him?" There are a couple of main donor banks. And we intentionally chose the European sperm bank, not UK.

Ria: You also have to consider what happens when the baby grows up. Our children would be able to contact the donor bank when they're older and then the donor bank would contact the donor. And similarly, there's a sibling list as well – there's a number attached to each child, as the sperm donor would have created various half siblings. So if our children wanted to find out if they had any siblings across the world, they could. That may all change, but that's as I understand it at the moment.

Fern: Importantly, the donors can only ever donate or give sperm to up to 10 families. It's not a huge number across the world, so that was a little bit reassuring – that we weren't using a donor who'd been used 100 times, or 500 times. And then you can go back to that particular donor and say, "I've had a donation from you previously and I'd like to extend the family. Would you consider giving more to us?"

Ria: We've also thought about how we talk to our children about it all. There's quite a bit of literature out there now for children. It's not going to be unusual, like when we grew up, so we'll be honest with them and we'll have that conversation with them and we will, fortunately, learn from our friends who've done it before us, and have told us what worked and what didn't work. We will always refer to 'the donor', though. It's never 'the dad'. I think there's still a lot of education that needs to be done around that, around what it means to us as parents and how we'd like people to talk about it.

Fern: And I think it is important to talk more openly about it and if people have questions, they just need to ask. And even close, close family – like our parents – sometimes just go, "Well, what happens here?" Or "Remind me of this part?" That's OK. You've just got to ask and there's not many people that are secretive about it. We've got to start saying, "Do you mind chatting about it?" I think that's only going to help in everyday language, such as preferring to call it a sperm donor.

Ria: I think what people should know too is that there are lots of challenges and hurdles with any fertility treatment – and there's a huge lack of control. I think when you're in a sporting environment, you think, 'I haven't quite done that, I just need to work on my strength' or 'I need to improve that aspect of my game.' There's no control in this situation and that's the thing that maybe I struggled with the most. For instance, in the sense that my eggs weren't maturing effectively when we first tried. That was hard. And then each stage, there's another conversation. Have they developed into blastocysts [the next stage of embryos]? And even then, you might be let down at the last minute for some reason if the embryos haven't done the right thing in the lab.

So if I could give any advice, then I would say: "Don't over-expect. Take each day as it comes and each step as it comes." In our case, we then had to go back to the hormone medication to try again. A huge setback. I was taking it to get my eggs ready and Fern was taking it to get her body ready for surrogacy.

Fern: We've had seven cycles of IVF in total to fall pregnant with our first child. I remember that cycle really hit us hard. There's always something, though. Another time, the transfer of the embryo goes well but you get a negative test two weeks later. We'd been so sure. We had sickness, we had sore boobs. Then you get a negative test. We also had one miscarriage. So we had a pregnancy test and we even got to the stage where we heard the heartbeat. But then we were told the baby wasn't growing as expected. That it was five days behind, I think it was. I miscarried around week 11. And you don't know what to expect. They give you options. Who knew they gave you options at miscarriage point? We got a pamphlet on each. I wanted my body to do it naturally rather than a tablet or surgery, though, and fortunately it did.

I think it would have helped if there was more support generally, though. I feel it would have helped me if I'd been able to talk to somebody about what to expect physically, for a start.

Ria: I felt useless. I underestimated the physical process of a miscarriage. I have major regrets in terms of my level of support for Fern, because I didn't know what would happen to her. After a period of time, what it did then was force a conversation about where we would go next. What would we do? I was thinking, 'Was my egg the problem, or is it Fern's oven?' They'd suggested it could be my egg so I did lots of things to change my diet, and I had acupuncture. I hate salmon and I was eating salmon twice a week because they said oily fish is good for you but actually it didn't work – none of it did. Without getting too religious, regardless of any diet, if it's going to work it's going to work. If it's not, it's not.

So it was then when we sat down and said, "Right, let's revisit this." And we decided to switch, didn't we? We would use Fern's eggs and I would carry. But for me, it was a really interesting time in my career because I was an interim Chief Executive and wanted to become full-time in that role. So there was a question about what I should do and how it would be perceived. And I think you then look at Jacinda Ardern, the former New Zealand Prime Minister – and I'm not comparing myself to her by any means! – but you look at someone like her, who's really open about how you can do both. You can have a career and be successful and be at the top of your game, *and* have a family. You can do them side by side. So we just did it, didn't we? Rather than put life on hold.

Once we'd decided that we would go again, then we bought a camper van and we got married and we went to Vegas. So actually, we just started living. And then maybe that made a difference to our mental health, which might be relevant – rather than putting yourself under pressure to give up the wine and the caffeine and eat food you don't like to eat. We enjoyed ourselves and then started the process again.

Fern: The next time around we were really enjoying the small wins. We've had some great eggs out. Yes, girl. Job done. That's a big tick in the box. Done. Next step. Don't get too excited. Don't get too disappointed. This is what it looks like. Because we knew every step, we felt more in control. I think that was a big one. We knew every single stage – and the moment we got that two-week test and then went to 6 weeks. And then you hear the heartbeat and you see it's the right size, and then we relaxed more at 20 weeks!

Ria: But I didn't want anyone to know. We didn't tell anybody and I said, "Don't tell my dad, because he'll be down in the pub telling everybody. So absolutely don't tell my dad." So then, over Christmas, we were then not drinking. So my brother was cottoning on, saying, "There's something not right here." But until we'd had that scan at 20 weeks, we were too nervous to say anything to anyone.

In the end, he came early – five weeks early. He was in intensive care for a couple of days, so that was another hurdle to get over – and it was during COVID.

It's also interesting because genetically it's Fern. I carried the pregnancy but it was Fern's eggs that we used. But then I try not to think about it too much:

biologically there's a connection because it's my blood, I carried him, it's my heartbeat. So I think I tried to hold on to that. There were times when he just wanted me as a baby too, because I was the one breastfeeding, so any fear about that connection went away. The fact that I've been part of the journey and I've carried – I was so fortunate. I'm so lucky that we've both been on the journey together and I've played a huge part. And he does some stuff – mainly his frown and his temper – and I know that's my boy!!

Fern: There are definitely some characteristics. Ria's laugh is very big and loud and he does that already. It's magical to see both of us in him. It is going to be really interesting next time because it's going to be my eggs in me. And there's going to be a natural link because we're using the same donor, which is going to be huge as well, and really important to us. Of course, there were all sorts of questions: did we really want the next baby to have the same donor? Did it matter? Because actually we're all growing up in one big family and we're all gonna do the same things and the house is gonna be full of love and full of laughter and probably full of music and sport. Perhaps it doesn't matter.

Ria: To anyone now embarking on a fertility journey, whether in a same-sex couple or not, I think you have to be pragmatic about the whole thing. It is what it is and that's the hardest thing, you know, with that control aspect. So, take the pressure off yourself, take each step as it comes to just try to be pragmatic about it. And if it's meant to be, it will be.

Fern: I think just go into it eyes wide open, and ask questions. And if you don't know what questions to ask, the one question you ask is, "What could go wrong at the next stage?" And you can then go into it with your eyes wide open. Continue to live your life, do things normally, do things that make you happy – continue that, continue life as much as possible, because mentally it will take over, naturally. And if you don't want to ask questions to the NHS or your private clinic, reach out to people who've gone through it and ask questions. I think that would be my best advice.

KEVIN & NICCI BUTTON

On male infertility

> **Kevin Button** founded *The Man Cave* after discovering he wasn't able to have children. When he and his wife **Nicci** appeared on my podcast, we discussed the largely taboo subject of male infertility. Kevin's diagnosis dramatically changed his outlook on life. Now, through social media, event organising and counselling, he's helping other men through their infertility challenges.
>
> 🎧 *Podcast released on 15 November 2020.*

Eight years ago, I found out I wasn't able to have children and it pretty much changed my life. To be honest, I didn't know how to take it. I was in denial for a while. I was in a bad place and my relationship broke down. The next thing I knew, I'd moved out and I was living with my dad. Later on, I got made redundant.

To go back to when I found out the news, I had a girlfriend at the time and we were trying for a baby. I think after about 12 to 14 months, we decided to go to the doctor's and I had a sperm sample taken. I had to do two in the end, and they were both showing low counts. I was advised to do a sperm retrieval operation. Again, they had no luck. It was heartbreaking.

My emotions were all over the place. I had no one to talk to, really, and it was a big struggle. There was no support out there. It was hard to try to talk to someone – frustration and anger would come out. Eventually, that meant my relationship broke down. However, then I met my wife, Nicci. And that's when we went on our fertility journey. We had two free cycles on the NHS, but we were unsuccessful. It was at that point that I started *The Man Cave*, which is all about spreading awareness around male infertility and its impacts on mental health.

I found that there was no one who could relate to my struggles because they hadn't been through the same process. And when I lost my cousin to suicide, that was life changing and I woke up one morning and decided I couldn't carry the burden around with me all the time. I had to get it off my chest and out. I made some close friends who were going through the same kind of thing and struggling and I just thought, 'I've got to do something about this.' I went on Instagram and I hadn't realised how big the 'trying to conceive' community was on there.

To be honest, I had many nights with my wife on the weekends when I would have a few beers and then I'd go to write posts, and then delete them. It just went on for many weeks, and then when my cousin passed away, I thought there was nothing to lose. I was 36 and I felt I had to help the other guys who were going through the same thing as me.

I reached out, and since then *The Man Cave* has been created and it's been growing stronger and stronger. I've been doing it for a while now, and a lot's happened. I think I've found my purpose. As soon as I started *The Man Cave*, it felt like a weight had been lifted and I feel much better now.

The real boss of all this, though, is my wife Nicci. She's just been amazing. She changed everything for me. When I got diagnosed – this was before Nicci – I went through the stages of meeting girls and when the topic of kids was brought up, I'd be quiet and then the next day, I'd send a message and say that children weren't for me. But that wasn't the case. I was scared. And then Nicci came along, and I did the same with her, funnily enough, and I said we should just be friends. A month later I dropped her a message and I told her everything, and she accepted me for who I was. It was pretty amazing for her to do that. We then went on our fertility journey.

We needed to go down the sperm donor route and it's been tough dealing with all the emotions, but the whole process has made us, as a couple, even stronger, because there were many points where we could have easily broken up.

There's hardly any support out there. People don't realise what you go through. It's a tough process – more needs to be done, and that's why I'm trying to educate people. First of all, I've educated myself about my own circumstances. With me, there is no sperm present. It's called azoospermia. They described it to me as having a factory, but no one is working. I remember waking up from the operation and the doctor gave me a letter. It basically said you've got two options: sperm donor and adoption. And then I went home.

From the perspective of a man struggling with fertility, I really have difficulty with conversations about children. People asking if we've got children. I avoid christenings and weddings, though I am trying to get better at that. I'm hoping by offering some support to people through

The Man Cave, I can help people like me feel less alone and get men to open up a bit.

There's a really concerning suicide rate amongst men of a certain age. It's the biggest killer of men under 45. And I'm really set on helping people who might feel like they are at rock bottom, because with infertility you go through some terrible emotions: anger and denial. You also struggle with stress and depression.

Nicci and I had counselling together – we had counselling for the first time for IVF problems. But some people don't feel they can talk to their partners, and it's hard to know where to turn. It's good on social media for some people as well, because they can remain anonymous if they want to. And I feel that a lot of men have been coming forward, speaking about their issues and their problems.

I'm on Twitter [@them_ancave] and Facebook [TheManCave], I've got my website [www.them-ancave.co.uk] and I do a lot of 'lives' on Instagram [them_ancave] too, and that's a massive community. It's helping me by helping others. I want to encourage more men to open up and talk and I also want to get support information into clinics as well. There needs to be something which helps men with the right information, rather than just a piece of paper like I had. There are men going through those doors every day.

It's also really tough to have those conversations with your partner about when might be the right time to stop. The *Man Cave* motto is 'Don't give up', but a lot of the time it does boil down to the financial side. We were lucky that we had two or three cycles on the NHS. And then we started to look at going abroad, but that'll only happen if I win a competition! As my friends know, I've got a bit of a reputation for winning competitions! The money, the failures – it's hard to deal with. Every cycle that doesn't work, you get more depressed. You try to be positive all the time, but then you go from one high to a big low and it's just tough, and it has an effect on your relationship. I tend to leave Nicci alone for a couple of weeks, give her some space and then talk it out, but I know couples find that hard. I think although we've found it hard, we believed we would just get stronger the more conversations we had.

When I was at my lowest was when I'd just had the diagnosis. To be honest, I was in denial for a while. I don't think it sank in until my relationship broke down with my girlfriend at the time. I was drinking heavily, I'm ashamed to say I was taking drugs at the time, and I was in a bad place. Then Nicci walked into my life and just changed everything.

Treatment then took over life, though. I think Nicci wanted to feel like she could have some kind of control, but couldn't, and I felt a bit helpless. I was trying to be supportive and positive all the time. I took up running. I took my frustration out on the pavement and though I hated running as a kid in school, for some reason, the last three or four years, I've done a lot of half marathons. And Nicci's doing well now too – she's done a Couch to 5K even though she suffers with asthma. The other factor is that you have to get your BMI down for fertility treatment – especially if we go abroad.

I'm starting to be more confident now and I feel like I've got a weight off my shoulders. I think I've got nothing to lose and I think that's due to maturity as well, the older I'm getting. I don't think 10 years ago I would have started *The Man Cave*, but the older you get, you suck it up and get it done. And yes, I'm much better now, I think.

NICCI BUTTON

One of my biggest worries has been my age. I'm 36 next month. So it's always sort of at the back of my mind. I'm also trying to keep fit and keep my weight down – taking up running and stuff to just try to help with the mental side as well. The last two goes we've not been successful and it's been rubbish. The second time was really good and we got to the transfer stage and that was really nice, but it's awful when you find out after the two-week wait that it hasn't worked – you tend to get your hopes up and get so excited.

Failing the second time was a lot harder than the first time. And then after our next go, it'll be down to money. I'm just so glad that Kev has *The Man Cave* to focus on. It's been amazing as before it felt so lonely, and just felt like I was failing when the IVF failed. I felt like I was the let-down. It's nice to have other people to connect to who understand, because as much as your family or friends want to, unless they've been there, they really can't.

My sister only had a baby 12 weeks ago. When they first found out this time last year that she was pregnant, there was this whole big thing with my family. I was upstairs working and I saw them outside of my mum's, all gathered at the bottom of the drive with my brother and his wife and her mum and my mum and my sister and her partner all getting together, and they shared the news and then nobody knew how to tell me. So then my mum pulled me aside, and it upset me so much. They didn't treat me normally. I thought, 'Why wouldn't you tell me? Why wouldn't I be happy?' But it was hard.

For us, at the end of the day, we know we want to be together. We've had the failures with IVF and we still know we want to be together, even though we might not have a family. We've made our commitment to each other. We know that even if it doesn't work next time, we still want to be together. It's not about having a baby because it's the next thing to do in life – it's because of the love you have for each other that you want to have a family, but I still want to share my life with Kev even if we don't have a baby.

I also try to remind myself that having a baby – you know, it's not all joyful and happy. As much as we want it desperately, that would be hard work and it puts a lot of strain on a relationship. I want to be with Kev even if it doesn't work. It wouldn't be the end of the world – well, maybe for a little while it would be, but not forever. We would pick ourselves up and move on together.

The first time we went through it, it was kept secret because we didn't want to share it, but I feel like it shouldn't be like that. And I feel like this time, since we've opened up, so many more people are talking about their struggles – how common they are. But on the whole, it's such a taboo subject and I just don't get why. Hopefully, as there is more and more stuff going out there about fertility journeys and about what people go through, it will become a bit more talked about and a bit more comfortable for people going through it. People should be able to feel they can express sadness and sorrow, as well as the joys.

DANIELLE BEATTIE

On recurrent miscarriage

> **Danielle Beattie** and I became friends through NCT (National Childbirth Trust) classes. Early on in our friendship, we discovered we had both experienced miscarriage before having our children. She was brave and open enough to talk to me about her and her husband Dylan's story, for which I will always be grateful. She also went on to take part in an award-winning documentary I made, called *Miscarriage: The Hidden Loss*, sensitively produced by Nicola Hendy.
>
> 🎧 *Podcast released on 3 February 2021.*

I've experienced three miscarriages whilst trying for our family.

We started trying to conceive, I think, around 2016. We were trying for 15 to 16 months. I have a history of polycystic ovaries, or polycystic ovary syndrome, so I had envisaged pregnancy being difficult, or getting pregnant being difficult. So it was no surprise to me that it had taken as long as it did.

When I first got pregnant in July 2017, we were overjoyed – but it was very short-lived. I found out on the Saturday that we were pregnant and by the Tuesday I was bleeding. So that was my first miscarriage and it was a spontaneous loss. I then got pregnant pretty much straight away and carried it until I was 13 weeks with that one. We'd had a private scan at 8 weeks because we were nervous, and we'd seen a heartbeat. We were approaching Christmas and all of our family were coming to stay, so we decided that we would announce on Christmas Day. However, we had a scan around 12 weeks on 18 December and we found that we'd lost that baby as well.

With the first miscarriage, I was quite pragmatic. I thought, 'Right, I can get pregnant. This isn't going to be impossible.' I had friends who had a history of miscarriage or not conceiving, so I felt very lucky to have fallen pregnant the first time, even though we'd lost the baby, because I felt like that gave me some hope. But the second one had a huge impact on me and my husband, simply because we'd built up that excitement the further we got along. What compounded that further was that the hospital said they couldn't do anything for us for another week because they have to see two scans a week apart without foetal activity, in case your dates are wrong. So, I went all the way through Christmas with that knowledge.

When it had been confirmed as a missed miscarriage, we chose to go with medical intervention. I had tablets, took them at home and then experienced the loss on 29 December. It was horrific. So painful. I mean, now that I've been through labour, I know that what I was experiencing was labour. My waters broke and then it was an entire horrific evening and whole next day of pain. It then took over a week for me to lose the afterbirth. All in all, the process lasted over three weeks. It was mental torture really, especially over the Christmas and New Year period, knowing that your body had failed you again – and then I felt like I'd failed my husband, because it was my body that was rejecting the pregnancy.

Then we were lucky enough to fall pregnant again later that year. And as a result of that, we've got Idris, who is an absolute crazy joy. Following that, though, I've had a third miscarriage this year. Again, I got to 12 weeks, but when I had the 12-week scan I found that everything had stopped growing at 7 weeks and it was another missed miscarriage.

This time I had the D&C, because I didn't want to go through the same thing as before with Idris being at home. I think I probably would have gone down the route of the tablets again had I not had a child at home, but you can't be unavailable when you've got a small child. So I went in and had the procedure and, of course, that in itself was so isolating because Dylan wasn't allowed to come in for any of the scans because of the pandemic. I had to do all that on my own. That's a brief history of my journey through pregnancy.

I'm now really apprehensive about trying again. We have decided that we will, but I'm 40 now so my age is against me. Obviously we have our ovarian reserve from birth, so my eggs are 40 years old – almost 41. I'm not certain whether miscarriage is more likely as I get older and I'm not sure that I can keep putting myself through it. I have discussed with Dylan that if it doesn't work this time then it will probably be the last, and that's scary because I don't really want Idris to be an only child. I've got two siblings – one older, one younger – and they can be a pain in the backside, but we're a crew! It was us with my mum, because my mum was a single parent. We were very tight-knit and when we lost our mum, I don't think I could have got through that without them, and that's why I really want a sibling for Idris. I want him to have that connection. So I'm apprehensive about the whole process, but at the same time, I want to give it just one more go. But then when does 'one more go' end? Because you do then think, 'Oh well, I'll give it one *more* try.' When do you stop? It's difficult. We didn't know exactly what might be causing the losses either. We would have had to experience a third pregnancy loss in a row before being referred for further testing. We had Idris so our miscarriages weren't consecutive.

It's really interesting how men deal with miscarriage too. With Dylan, my husband, when we speak about pregnancy, he automatically says, "when you were pregnant", and that's correct. I'm pregnant – *we're* not pregnant, *I* was pregnant. But when he talks about loss, he says "we", and always has: "when we lost". And I wasn't sure with Dylan whether that was a conscious, 'I'm not blaming *you*' terminology. So we had a discussion about it on a car journey and he said, "No, it's because: yes, *you're* pregnant, but *we* lose those babies, that's *our* loss." So he said, no, it's not a conscious change of vocab for him. It just is, *we* experienced the loss. "Even though it was only *you* that was pregnant, they were *our* children, or would have been our children, they were *our* babies." So it is quite interesting that he thinks like that. Because men do get left out of the loop. They're meant to be the strong ones to support you.

I found, when we were in hospital, I hadn't noticed anyone asking Dylan if he was okay. When we've had that news, and when we've been going through things, I don't think anything has ever been directed towards him. And we're *both* going through it. It's not necessarily the case that the men should have to be strong for us, because *their* dreams are crumbling right in front of them as well. For him, it was a huge loss as well. Just as it was for me, but he wasn't getting that care.

I wish I could give advice, but it's so individual. It's such an individual experience, so it depends on how you as a person take it. I suppose the only thing I would say is: don't give up hope, because many, many people will experience a lot of loss and will go on to have children. And also, there is life outside children as well. It may not be what people will want to hear if they're really trying, but I have friends who have tried and failed to have a child and they've found happiness in other areas. I mean, I suppose the one thing that I always kept in mind was that I was very happy in my marriage and as much as we wanted our baby, who we now have, we would have been happy without him too.

Also, keep the dialogue going with your partner. Don't ever shut them out, because they're probably feeling exactly the same way that you are. They're just not going through it physically. And watching you go through it physically is going to be really painful for them. Obviously not physically painful, but as emotionally painful. I suppose that's given us the strength to carry on through the loss.

STEPHEN ASHE & TERESA COOTES

On surrogacy in the UK

> **Stephen Ashe** and his male partner have two children, both born using surrogates. Stephen went on to become a client manager for surrogacy agency Brilliant Beginnings. He spoke about his experience as an 'intended parent' – the term used for parents awaiting a baby being carried by a surrogate. He was also speaking in his role at the agency at the time, where he matched intended parents with surrogates and helped them to navigate their journey.
>
> **Teresa Cootes** was a surrogate mum. She worked with Brilliant Beginnings and spoke of her experience of carrying children for others, the challenges of the process and the immense satisfaction she got from it.
>
> 🎧 *Podcast released on 13 March 2021.*

Stephen: My surrogacy experience is through having two children of my own, through surrogacy. My partner and I are gay. We always knew that we wanted to have children but that we wouldn't be able to do that in the normal way. And we were really amazed and excited to find out about surrogacy many years ago, and pursued a journey through surrogacy in the UK, and have a 5 and a 7 year old now. I'm really excited because, as well as my personal experience of surrogacy and being a parent through surrogacy, I've since had the opportunity to work at Brilliant Beginnings as a Client Manager, and that's really helped me to be able to pass on my own experience and help other intended parents go through their own surrogacy journeys.

Teresa: I started thinking about becoming a surrogate way back probably in 2013, when I'd originally offered to help one of my siblings who was struggling to conceive. But, happily, they didn't actually need my help and managed to carry their own children. But the idea of helping somebody stuck with me. So I spent a lot of time researching what surrogacy was, making sure that I felt informed about what I was getting myself into – and because I have my own children as well, so I wanted to be confident that this was something I could do. And then I started looking specifically at different organisations in the UK that could possibly help me with that. I did my first journey and delivered twins, a boy and a girl, back in October 2017, so they're now 3 years old. I'm currently on my second journey with a new couple of intended parents, and I'm in the early stages of a pregnancy for them as well.

Stephen: It is possible to do surrogacy in the UK. The negative is that there just aren't enough surrogates coming forward for the number of intended parents that are looking. Intended parents need to make their decisions based on the fact that they might be waiting for some time. It is also the case that many of the intended parents that I speak to have considered friends or family, and that's an amazing route for surrogacy as well.

All of our teams at Brilliant Beginnings bring together an agreement, and although it's not legally enforceable in the UK, it is massively important to have explored all the different eventualities and what everyone's expectations are. I think for friends or family members, where the intended parent and surrogate already know each other, it's even more important to have that sort of third party help to navigate some of those really tough conversations. When it's someone that you know really well, that you have an existing relationship with, those can be very difficult to have.

Teresa: I'm not a lawyer. I don't have a legal brain. There were lots of things that I knew would come up in the journey. I wouldn't know how to begin even having those discussions, and how would I find intended parents? So that was a massive driving factor for me. Finding an organisation that could provide that support was a really, really big relief for me. It's the thought, as well, that we are so blessed to have our own children – and all surrogates will have had their own children: that's one of the criteria in the UK. And so we know the joy that they bring, we know how amazing it is to be able to have a family to love. And having had good pregnancies myself (and lots of surrogates that I know have had good pregnancies and good labours), it feels like a very small thing that we can do to extend to somebody else, to give them that lifetime of happiness and that family that we treasure so much.

Stephen: We want to keep the numbers of surrogates that are coming through and inquiring and progressing through screening and preparation with our Surrogate Managers at a quite sensible ratio to the number of intended parents that are waiting. So we're constantly reviewing that. Our aim is to match one-to-one. They're surrogates and intended parents that are aligned on things like personality as much as some of the bigger things, like views on termination.

Teresa: I think as a surrogate going through it – and I've gone through it now twice, with two different couples for two different journeys – I've always taken great comfort in the match that would be made for me being the best match, but fundamentally the aim was always to avoid any kind of discontent or breakdown in relationships or anything like that. So I always felt very confident that those key things in the agreements, about how I would give birth or where I would give birth, which were quite important to me, would all be discussed well ahead of time, and that I would only ever be matched with intended parents that either aligned with me perfectly on those key issues or were at least open to having those discussions. Because, obviously, it would make no sense if you were matched with people that had very opposing views on some of those key things. And then I think it was very nice that, actually, I found that with the two couples that I've been matched with, we have coincidentally had things in common. It allowed for us to have a much more organic and natural bond, and a friendship that developed.

One of the most common questions that I get from others interested in being surrogates is "What will happen if the parents change their mind? What will happen if I'm left holding the baby?" Equally, intended parents worry that the surrogate will change her mind as well. And so a lot of the work and a lot of the discussions that we find ourselves having are to reassure them that while the law is really clunky and very outdated, there are things that can be put in place, that we do put in place. That there is a pathway that they can follow that will really minimise that risk and make it almost non-existent, and that there are safeguarding measures put in place on both sides.

Stephen: In terms of UK surrogate expenses, the way it works at Brilliant Beginnings is that the Surrogate Managers will be sitting down with the surrogates that are coming through screening and preparation from the outset to talk about these things, and expenses can look different for different people. So the range that we see [in March 2021] is between £12,000 at the lower end and £20,000 at the upper end. And because a surrogate should not be out of pocket, it does mean different things for different people.

The clinical side will vary depending on whether intended parents have been through an IVF journey and have managed to create embryos already. Clearly the costs will be less in that case, and it will be about preparing the surrogate for an embryo transfer and the clinical costs for that. Others may be coming to this needing the help of an egg donor, needing to create embryos, so the costs around that will be higher. We also say to intended parents, really you should be anticipating that the first transfer may not work, so you ought to be budgeting for a couple of transfers. We hope that in creating embryos, you'll have enough embryos to transfer and it won't be a question of going back to the beginning again. From a health perspective, once the pregnancy has been established, we have the advantage of the NHS here, which is fantastic and free at the point of use for our surrogates when they give birth.

There are legal costs, obviously. The legal side really depends on how much time you want to put into this and how quickly you want the legal process to be resolved. So that is clearly going to happen more quickly, and with less effort on the intended parents' part, if you have the help of an organisation to help you through that. And particularly at the moment with parental orders, what we're seeing with intended parents that are choosing a surrogate in the UK for a UK birth, if they're deciding to run that process themselves, is that it can take nine to twelve months after the baby is born for you to have that parental order issued and to have a birth certificate. If you're having help coordinating that, it can come down to six months, even less. For many intended parents, you want that resolved as soon as possible.

Going back to budget, if you're looking for help from a full-service support agency like Brilliant Beginnings and you need to create embryos, cover the costs and have help on the legal side, in terms of a sort of ballpark figure, I think intended parents should have in mind a range of £50,000 to £60,000 in the UK [in March 2021].

Teresa: One of the great things is the bond and the friendships that I have created with my intended parents. With my first journey, that's continued beyond the delivery of the twins, and we are still in each other's lives in a very realistic way, being that we now all have children and jobs and stuff like that. And that's really nice: you can't ever have too many people loving a child or caring about the welfare of that child. But other really key amazing things to be able to witness as a surrogate are the joy on the faces of the parents when they hear that the IVF has worked and you are pregnant; the first time they see the heartbeat; and seeing them anticipate the arrival of this baby. For a lot of couples and a lot of single intended parents coming to surrogacy now, there will have been a time in their lives when they thought that those things would never happen for them.

I haven't met a surrogate yet who wouldn't like to have a cuddle at some point after the delivery, to be able to say hello to this little person that they've been growing for nine months. But it is so important for us to be able to see the parents have that moment as well – and lots and lots of surrogates, as they come through screening, are really adamant: the parents should absolutely be holding that baby first. Early skin to skin, let them be in the room, and let them see this happening. For us, that doesn't feel strange at all. It feels natural that they should be there. This is their pregnancy, this is their child coming into the world. When you know that these people have really gone through a journey and how much it's meant to them, and that it was possible in no small part because of you, that is a really delicious feeling. I won't lie.

And then also, beyond the delivery, it's important to agree on what kind of relationship you want to have. How much do you want to be involved in this child's life and want them to know about you? And that forms part of that matching criteria as well. Obviously, you wouldn't match intended parents who wanted an ongoing relationship with a surrogate who felt actually she wanted very much to get back to her own children. So those are things that we align on as well. We obviously encourage the relationship to continue. It's very good for babies born through surrogacy to know about where they've come from. I know from my experience, the twins that I delivered have two dads. And so even at 3 years old, they're coming to a point where they have questions about how come their family looks slightly different to some of the other children they know in nursery. And so it's good for parents to be able to have those open conversations. And we also find, as well, that in these kinds of circumstances, if the adults in the lives of the children are very open about what's going on and their conversations are very positive, then the children will reflect that. That's what they will take away from that experience.

Stephen: The highlights of the surrogacy experience for me as an intended parent were definitely sharing those moments with our surrogates and having the opportunity to attend the embryo transfer. And as the pregnancies progressed, we went along to scans, we met up for lunch. They're amazing experiences. And the relationships that we built during that time, they'll last forever. I think one thing that stood out for me around the birth was that surrogates want to help create families. When my son was born, my mum had the opportunity to visit the hospital quite soon after. And I remember we were all in the same room: myself, my partner, the surrogate, our son, and my mum. My mum was holding our son, and she just couldn't express enough thanks to our surrogate about making her a grandmother. And it's about grandmothers as well. There are other people involved in this. And I could see on our surrogate's face that, for her, that was just an amazing thing to hear.

Teresa: I think something else that I really value, and hopefully other surrogates are valuing as well, is the surrogate community that we're building – with other women that are either in a surrogate journey, have had a surrogacy journey, or are thinking very seriously about whether this is right for them. And being able to connect and talk with other women in a safe space, in a positive way. It's a supportive environment where women can feel open to ask questions, where we can congratulate each other and celebrate the little milestones that come along as well. And that – for me, definitely, and I know for other surrogates – has been really amazing.

I think if I could say one thing to anybody thinking about coming to surrogacy, whether that's as an intended parent or as a surrogate themselves, it would be: this is a life-changing experience. You wouldn't buy a house without having the proper support – surveyors, solicitors in place, mortgage brokers and things like that – to make sure that everything went smoothly. Comparing these two things as significant life experiences, taking on the support of professionals in the fertility world and in the surrogacy industry that can support you through that is a very natural response to have, for me, and to have that responsibility largely taken out of my hands.

Stephen: I would always say to people from the very beginning to bear in mind that this is going to take a while. It is an amazing journey to be on, but it could take quite a while. A lot of couples think that once they've got embryos and a surrogate, that's it. That's a good place to be at, but there are some other things that have to happen as well for you to get to the point of coming home with a baby. And for me as an intended parent, managing those expectations was key, but also realising that until you're holding that baby in your arms, there's always going to be a little bit of a niggling doubt in your mind: 'Is this really going to happen for me?' And it will, but it will take time.

GABBY LOGAN

Reflecting on fertility treatment

> **Gabby Logan** is a well-known sports broadcaster, married to former rugby International Kenny Logan. She joined me on the podcast to discuss her experience with IVF and look back on what it felt like then, and what it means now. Gabby and Kenny have twins, Reuben and Lois.
>
> 🎧 *Podcast released on 26 September 2021.*

Although it's now more than 15 years ago, I can tap back into the memories of our IVF experience quite quickly. It happened over a long period of time, it's life changing and it stays with you. So I have a lot of internal conversations about it.

To go back to the beginning, when I first realised there might be a problem: I was about 28 and we had married in the July. A few months later I remember telling some girlfriends when we were out that I wanted to start trying to have a family. They were all about the same age, and they seemed shocked, I remember, because of my career focus. I remember that as the point at which I was starting to think about getting pregnant.

From then, about a year passed, and I realised that I wasn't pregnant. I was thinking, 'That's strange,' but I wasn't panicking because Kenny was playing rugby, we were busy, and there was nothing fundamentally wrong with my cycle. I'd never had endometriosis or polyps or anything like that. I'd just had normal periods my whole life, hardly ever been on the pill, and only temporarily been on the coil. I felt quite normal. My mum had had four kids, everybody else in our family had multiple children.

Then six months after that, I remember Kenny was playing for Scotland and I was in Edinburgh and I walked into a Waterstones and I just found myself in the mother and baby section. Suddenly, I found myself pulling a book out about fertility, and it's the first time I'd done any serious thinking about it. I remember crouching down in the corner of Waterstones hoping nobody would see me reading this book about fertility, and having the realisation that I had passed all these milestones that it was talking about. It said things like, 'if you're not pregnant within the first year...', for instance.

I was 29 then, but I still didn't panic at that point, even though the alarm bells started ringing. I just thought, 'We'll just have to be a bit more dedicated to the cause.' I started noticing my cycle more, such as noting when I might be ovulating, because I hadn't really thought about any of those things.

I had a good friend whose husband played rugby with Kenny, for Wasps, and she used to get pregnant like shelling peas. She'd pee on an ovulation stick and then she'd be pregnant, so gradually I realised that maybe we had an issue. As time went on, we went to see a gynaecologist and that's when it really started to ramp up a bit. He was saying, "You've gone two years now, you know?", and he did the dye through the tubes [HSG] and all of that stuff.

Making Babies podcast: Gabby Logan

That procedure was really uncomfortable and I remember going to a friend's birthday and feeling like I'd been punched in the stomach. At that point it felt like it had all got quite medical quite quickly. But I still felt that we'd go back to see the gynaecologist and he would give a straightforward diagnosis and a pill to fix it and it would all be fine. I was even thinking, "Maybe he'll discover a baby in the meantime!"

Instead he said, "There's nothing wrong. Your tubes are fine and you're having periods." And, of course, Kenny had also had all the tests on his sperm and motility was fine, numbers were fine. So we were a bit deflated not to get any answers.

The gynaecologist said we had plenty of time as we were still young. But we didn't really want to hear that, because we realised that this was going to become a big thing. Plus, I knew that Kenny was really keen to have a family at a younger age, because his dad had died when he was 19. His dad had him at 50 and it was really important to Kenny that he didn't want his kids to lose him in the way he lost his dad. So he was so supportive of whatever I wanted to do – he would support it in any way. And IVF was one of those options. I said to Kenny, "We'll never know what's wrong until we actually get some kind of embryo under a microscope. We'll be wondering if your sperm and my eggs just never want to get together." I thought then at least we'd know if we may need to have an egg donor or a sperm donor.

I had a friend who was adopted, and later had cancer. She was desperate to have her own family because she'd been adopted, but she was told not to get pregnant because of her cancer – but she defied it, went to America and had an egg donor and had two children. I remember thinking that we might have to have an egg donor. I just didn't know enough about it at all and I hadn't heard many conversations about it.

It was very isolating. People just didn't talk as much then. Social media wasn't the same. Fifteen years ago, there was barely Twitter and even if there had been, people would never have discussed something like this. There wouldn't have been an account that was about fertility. My mum had four children very easily in her early twenties and then my brother was a lot later in her thirties, so I didn't really want to start talking to my wider family. I thought, 'If this is going to be something that's going to take a very long time, I don't want to become that person that only ever talks about this. I don't want it to define me.'

For example, before IVF had actually begun for us, we'd gone to a wedding. The bride's mother said to me as she looked at a baby who was there, "but you're such a career woman," or something similar – as if a baby wasn't for me. And there were several other comments like that, implying that I'd made a decision not to have children – especially as we'd got a dog by this point, as we'd also been told that dogs encourage the right hormones! I think people started assuming we were dog people and that was that.

It wasn't just a dog we tried. I was having acupuncture. I'd been having acupuncture for years anyway, and my acupuncturist was really very natural and all about the five elements in Chinese medicine. I'm someone who believes in the science of things, but also in alternatives. I like a balance. But eventually we did accept that IVF was a path well-trodden and it may just be something we had to do.

In the end I said to Kenny, "Look, I think we just go for it because that's the only way we're going to know. If we're going to need five rounds, six rounds, it's better to get started." In total, it was probably three years from starting trying naturally to actually having IVF.

At that point Kenny was in the last year of his playing career and he'd decided to play for Glasgow for a season. We still had our house in London and then we had an apartment in Glasgow. He was flying back and forth a lot. I was doing the Champions League for ITV and I remember not only being apart from Kenny a lot as we started treatment, but also being very busy with work, and I was going through airports with my little bag of drugs and stuff. I went and paid a visit to my mum once, because I was doing a Man United game and she's in Leeds, and I remember putting them on this window sill outside. It was November and I had to keep them cold and do my injections and I remember her knocking on my bedroom door as I was about to do an injection – but I didn't even want her to know at that stage. My parents were going through a divorce and she was having a really hard time so I didn't want to add stress, plus I was conscious that it might not work.

I think, overall, maybe we treated it a bit like sportspeople might. This is the schedule, this is what we've got to do, it's going to take this amount of time and this is the end aim – but still, when I look back, I do see times when it did get more emotional. For example, when we reached nearer the end – when we got to harvesting of the eggs and fertilisation and then the nervous wait to see whether they'd made it to the blastocyst stage. And then waiting for the transfer date to be set. And then the transfer itself.

I don't know how many days later it would have been, when I was supposed to be going to get my blood test after the embryo transfer, but I bled that morning before the test and decided that was it – I definitely wasn't having a baby. I was really upset and Kenny was in Glasgow at the time, so he wasn't even able to come with me. However, the doctor said, "Let's just get the blood test done anyway." We found out we were pregnant. So it hadn't been a miscarriage.

Support throughout the process was difficult. My very best friend had her eldest (who I'm godparent to) two years earlier by accident and then just before I started IVF, she had twins naturally. I just felt as if I couldn't tell her as I didn't think she'd get it, and when I did eventually tell her, she didn't know what IVF was. She didn't know whether they were my babies, so I had to explain a lot. But that's just because she'd never been anywhere near it as a conversation.

Overall, I think Kenny was enough support for me. The conversations we were able to have were enough. It was our journey together and he was so supportive. That was sufficient, along with the medical support. I had a great gynaecologist and even Bill, who did my scans, I can still see him in my mind's eye. He was always laughing and joking. He had such a nice way about him and he often had to give good – and bad – news to people. The clinic itself wasn't daunting for me as I saw it as a place where good stuff was going to happen. I had a really positive vibe about it. It was only on the day when I went to my

Making Babies podcast: Gabby Logan

blood test and I was bleeding that I'd actually entertained the idea that I was potentially not going to have a baby.

Kenny didn't seek other support either as this was happening. However, before we got married, he had a full medical, regarding his sperm, because he was concerned about being kicked quite a lot down there because of rugby. He told me later that he didn't want to propose to me and then find out he was infertile. He was fine according to all the tests, but overall there was never a sense of anyone being to blame when it came to needing treatment. It was just something we were going through together, even though it was happening physically to me and not to him. I do think maybe there was some guilt that he wasn't having any of the physical changes. He wasn't having to inject himself. He wasn't having to dash around to get a blood test. But he was always supportive.

Luckily for him, one of the fitness coaches at his club was a really good friend and he was able to ask quietly for the odd day off to do something. He didn't say what it was, but the funny thing was, they later came and spoke to us because they went through IVF years later.

I also remember that Kenny used to come up with some amusing comparisons. Having a farming background, and having a dad and brother who were world-renowned inseminators, he used to draw parallels with livestock! I was very clear that I wasn't having his family involved in any way in that process! But actually we needed some of this banter to help lighten the atmosphere at times.

Going back to the transfer, I should say we went for the option of putting two embryos back. At that point, one child was more than we had been daring to dream about.

Then unbelievably, at the scan at around 8 weeks, there were two heartbeats. The doctor had said something to me when he read the blood tests about levels being high but I hadn't picked up on it and all I heard was that I was pregnant. We still didn't tell anyone, though, and even when we did tell my mum at Christmas, we still didn't say that it was twins. We did relax a bit more after the 12-week scan, and then I did start focusing on the twin pregnancy.

It feels like a long pregnancy when you go through IVF, because you start so far in advance with planning the treatment and there's no element of surprise. I've had friends that found out they were pregnant at 16 weeks and then only had 20 weeks until they gave birth. It felt like I was pregnant for a long time.

When we did eventually tell my family, they were very surprised and I think my mum did wonder why I hadn't spoken to her about it. But it wasn't going to take away from the joy. I gradually explained it all to more family and friends, and I think many people realised they were lucky to get pregnant so easily.

Amongst Kenny's teammates at Wasps, there were a few of us who were really good friends and people did begin to talk later on, and we realised that no journey is straightforward. One of my friends told me she'd had a tumour growing with one pregnancy and it had to be taken out at five months and the baby could have died. That had been happening around the same time as we were going through treatment and we had no idea. Another couple that we knew had also had fertility issues, it turned out later. It's very rarely without any issues at all for people.

Making Babies podcast: Gabby Logan

Fast forward a bit, and then we had to make another decision. We had five embryos 'on ice'. In the back of our minds, I think we thought the original problem might have been sorted out now that I'd already managed to fall pregnant once, so we thought we might fall pregnant naturally at some stage. First of all we spent a few years simply living in chaos with twins, thinking when life returned to normal, we'd think about another child. But, of course, it never does get back to normal and although I never went back on contraception, we never fell pregnant again after Lois and Reuben.

I'll never really know the reasons we could never seem to fall pregnant naturally, but about six months ago, I was interviewing somebody for my podcast *The Mid·Point*. She was a doctor and she said to me when we were off the podcast that there are these little hairs in our tubes that kind of help push the eggs down. She thought it may have been my issue and she explained that nowadays that can be rectified.

Overall, though, we felt very lucky to have had two healthy babies and at that point, we didn't want to push our luck. At the ten-year point after the treatment, we did have to have a really honest conversation, because that's when legally the stored embryos were supposed to not be kept anymore. We walked around to a local pub and had lunch together, and I said I was really up for it, but Kenny felt that we had two healthy children and he was a bit nervous about me. He worried that it might change me, especially as I'd had quite a traumatic birth – something he had more memories of than me.

My feeling was that I was frustrated that I had to choose whether to use the embryos, because what I'd

209

really wanted was to fall pregnant naturally. I felt my body had done it once. So in the end we made the choice not to use them. We were lucky, too, because we already had a boy and a girl.

When the twins were about 12, they started doing sex education at school. Once they understood reproduction, I wanted them to know how they came about. But when we told them, their reaction was strange – as if they couldn't believe it, and maybe the next minute I was going to tell them they were adopted or something. They were very dramatic about it, but then they decided to tell some friends and when they realised they weren't bothered, the twins became very relaxed about it too. After all, it's not dramatic: you just came about a slightly different way. And when kids throw that line back to their parents – "Why did you even have me in the first place?" then I can say, "You can never tell me that I didn't want you because I absolutely *did* want you." We wanted them so badly, we had to do it another way.

I've also talked to my daughter about infertility and we've had a conversation about whether it means she'll have problems. I said that there's no reason why she should, but there's no guarantee either. If you look at my mum's mum, she had four children and my sisters and brothers have all had children. Nobody else in our family has gone through IVF, but I also said to remember she could be the most fertile person in the world – so don't take any risks!

On my podcast I also talk about hormones at the other end of fertility. We address the menopause and it's been interesting to look at hormones and our bodies later on. I think actually IVF has helped me address my own menopause. I think some women feel a barrenness when their periods stop and there's a sudden psychological barrier to moving through the menopause. I don't quite feel that. My doctor thought I'd be concerned when she told me my hormone blood levels, but I was really OK with them and the fact I'd be going through menopause. I think probably because of what we'd been through, it wasn't quite as traumatic an idea for me.

I feel at peace with that and I feel at peace with not having tried again with the frozen embryos now – although there's always that twinge. For instance, when my colleague Denise Lewis had a baby at I think 46, I did feel clucky, but I'm at peace with it now.

Glossary of technical terms

anti-Müllerian hormone (AMH) test: This is a straightforward blood test. AMH plays a key role in developing a foetus' sex organs, and AMH levels correspond to the number of eggs you have in your ovaries, with higher levels meaning more eggs. The test may also show how well you respond to fertility drugs aimed at stimulating your ovaries to mature multiple eggs in preparation for IVF.

azoospermia: This is when there are no sperm in the man's ejaculate. This can be because of a blockage, or due to decreased sperm production. Around 10% of infertile men and 1% of all men have azoospermia.

blastocyst: A ball of cells that forms very early in a pregnancy, about five to six days after a sperm fertilises an egg. It implants in your womb lining, eventually becoming the embryo and then the foetus.

cervix: The lower, narrow end of the uterus (womb), which connects it to the vagina. Menstrual blood passes through it from the uterus into the vagina, and the strongest sperm pass through it in the other direction to fertilise eggs. It widens during the birth of a baby.

chemical pregnancy: A very early pregnancy loss, before the fifth week. Some women may not even realise they have experienced a chemical pregnancy as they might not have missed their period.

Glossary of technical terms

Clexane: An anticoagulant drug. It stops unwanted blood clots from forming and can stop any blood clots that have already formed from growing bigger.

cytokines: Proteins in your body which help control inflammation. They tell immune cells where to go and what to do to keep your immune system functioning correctly, to defend your body against germs or other substances that could make you ill. Too many cytokines can cause excess inflammation and conditions like autoimmune diseases.

dilation and curettage (D&C): A procedure to remove tissue from inside your uterus (womb). Performed to diagnose and treat certain conditions in the uterus, such as heavy bleeding, or to remove the womb lining after a miscarriage or abortion.

doxycycline: An antibiotic usually used to treat infections caused by bacteria, such as chest and dental infections, skin conditions and sexually transmitted infections. It can also be used to prevent malaria.

drug protocol: This is a combination of drugs which are prescribed together as if they were one thing.

egg / ovum: The ovum/egg cell is produced by a woman's reproductive system. Women begin puberty with about 300,000 to 400,000 eggs already inside their ovaries.

egg collection / egg retrieval: The procedure to collect the eggs from one or both ovaries. It takes place under anaesthetic.

embryo: An offspring in the early stages of development, in particular a human offspring from approximately the second to the eighth week after fertilisation (after which it is usually called a **foetus**).

embryo transfer: A few days after the eggs are collected and then fertilised, the embryos are transferred into the womb. This is done using a thin tube called a **catheter**, which is passed into your vagina.

endometritis: Inflammation of the lining of the uterus, caused by an infection. (NB Not to be confused with **endometriosis**, where tissue similar to the womb lining grows in other places, e.g. the ovaries and fallopian tubes.)

endometrium: The lining of the uterus. The body prepares this during the menstrual cycle, in order to host an embryo.

fallopian tubes: The two tubes in a woman's body which eggs released by the ovaries travel through to get to the womb.

foetus: A developing offspring in the womb, from around the eighth week after fertilisation until birth.

follicle: A follicle is a small sac of fluid in the ovaries that contains a developing egg. During each monthly menstrual cycle a number of follicles, each containing an egg, grow and mature.

frozen embryo transfer (FET): When an embryo that was created on a previous cycle of IVF treatment is thawed and transferred into the womb.

gestational carrier: Another term for a surrogate.

granulocyte colony-stimulating factor (G-CSF): This helps to increase the blood supply to the womb lining and the regeneration of its cells. It may increase the chances of the embryo being successfully implanted into the womb lining and staying there during the pregnancy.

Glossary of technical terms

human chorionic gonadotropin (HCG): The hormone you produce during pregnancy, which is also often administered as a 'trigger' injection in the final stage of an IVF cycle. This prompts all the follicles which have grown eggs to release them in one go, to be collected in the egg-harvesting procedure.

Humira: A drug injected under your skin to reduce inflammation by blocking part of your immune system.

hysterosalpingogram (HSG): An examination where dye is injected so that the inside of your uterus (womb) and fallopian tubes can be seen more clearly via X-ray.

hysteroscopy: Procedure with a small camera which allows a surgeon to look inside your uterus (womb) in order to diagnose and treat causes of abnormal bleeding, like polyps or fibroids.

intended parents: Individuals who enter into an agreement to become the parents of a child born to a surrogate.

intracytoplasmic sperm injection (ICSI): A technique used during IVF where a single sperm is injected directly into an egg for the purpose of fertilisation.

intralipid infusion: An intravenous infusion to provide essential fatty acids that it's thought could be helpful for women who have suffered repeat miscarriages. It is normally given once or twice prior to the pregnancy and then once per month after the initial conception attempt.

intrauterine insemination (IUI): The procedure when a sperm sample that has been given and frozen is thawed and inserted into the uterus.

in vitro fertilisation (IVF): The process where mature eggs are collected from ovaries and fertilised by sperm in a lab, and the resulting embryos implanted back into the uterus. One full cycle of IVF normally takes from three to six weeks.

karyotype test: A check of the chromosomes inside cells to see if anything is unusual. The test may be done on the fluid from the amniotic sac containing a developing baby, in order to spot abnormalities, or on would-be parents who are having fertility issues, to find out whether there is a chromosome problem.

laparoscopy: Often performed on women with unexplained infertility, this is an operation where a thin lighted tube is inserted into a tiny incision in your abdomen and sends video images to a computer screen. It can also be used to do a biopsy of suspect growths that may be hampering fertility.

magnetic resonance imaging (MRI): A type of diagnostic test using magnets and radio waves to create detailed images of organs, bones, muscles and blood vessels.

miscarriage: The spontaneous loss of a foetus before the end of the 24th week of pregnancy. Pregnancy losses after that stage are called **stillbirths**.

missed miscarriage: A missed (or silent) miscarriage is one where the embryo or foetus has died, but has remained in the womb. In many cases, there has been no sign that anything was wrong, so the news can come as a complete shock.

myomectomy: Surgery to remove fibroids from the uterus, leaving the uterus intact so pregnancy is still possible.

Glossary of technical terms

The National Institute for Health and Care Excellence (NICE): A public sector organisation which assists the UK government by publishing healthcare guidelines for the NHS in Wales and England.

natural killer cells: These are white blood cells which destroy infected cells and cancer cells in the body as part of the immune system. Some women have an immune disorder which causes their natural killer (NK) cells to attack the developing embryo.

oestrogen: One of the main female sex hormones. It is needed for puberty, the menstrual cycle, pregnancy, bone strength and other functions of the body.

ovulation: The process in which an egg is released from an ovary.

ovulation window: The time during your menstrual cycle when you're most likely to get pregnant. For most women, this lasts seven days: the five days leading up to ovulation (which occurs about 12–14 days before your period starts), the day of ovulation and the day after ovulation.

ovum: See *egg / ovum*.

parental order: This transfers legal parenthood of a baby born through surrogacy from the surrogate (and her spouse or civil partner if she has one) to the intended parent(s) – the intended parent(s) will need to apply to the court to have it awarded.

polycystic ovary syndrome (PCOS): A problem with hormones that can happen during a woman's reproductive years. PCOS sufferers may not have periods very often, or may have periods that last many days. They may also have too much of a 'male' hormone called androgen. This condition may lead to difficulty in getting pregnant as eggs are often not released.

polyp: In the uterus, this is a projecting growth of the womb lining. Large ones can cause infertility or miscarriage.

preimplantation genetic screening (PGS): This is when embryos which may look perfectly healthy under a microscope are tested for underlying chromosomal defects before being transferred into the womb.

progesterone: A hormone that helps create a healthy womb lining to maintain a pregnancy. Low levels can cause complications such as bleeding or miscarriage.

prolactin: A hormone responsible for certain breast tissue development and milk production.

prolactinoma: A noncancerous tumour of the pituitary gland which causes it to make too much prolactin. The main effect is decreased levels of oestrogen and testosterone, and it can cause decreased libido, impotence in men, abnormal milk flow or menstruation problems in women, and infertility.

speculum: A medical tool for investigating body orifices. It is inserted, for example, into the vagina during a routine smear test.

sperm: Produced in the testicles, the head of the sperm carries the DNA which enables it to create a new individual when combined with the DNA in a woman's egg. Sperm can live inside the female reproductive tract for about three to five days after sex.

stillbirth: When a foetus dies in the 25th week of pregnancy or later, either in the womb or during birth.

Glossary of technical terms

surrogacy: When a woman carries and gives birth to a baby for another person or couple.

Tamoxifen: A drug used to treat and prevent breast cancer. A selective oestrogen receptor modulator (SERM – oestrogen is known as estrogen in the US), it may also initially stimulate ovulation and increase fertility.

trigger injection: See *human chorionic gonadotropin*.

transvaginal ultrasound: A relatively quick, painless imaging procedure used to diagnose conditions affecting the female reproductive organs or to monitor a pregnancy. With the probe inserted into the vagina, it provides a more detailed view than an external ultrasound.

uterine embolization: A procedure to shrink fibroids in the uterus by blocking their blood supply.

uterus: The medical term for the womb.

Acknowledgements

THE EXPRESSION 'AN emotional rollercoaster' gets overused, but in the case of writing this book, every feeling has emerged at some point or another.

If anyone knows the animated film *Inside Out*, you'll know what I mean when I say that 'Joy', 'Sadness', 'Fear', 'Anger' and 'Disgust' were all working overtime in my hive of a brain as I tried to process all the events of the past decade. With the tangled messiness of life thrown in alongside the many twists and turns we were destined to make to start a family, it was perhaps a foolish idea to relive all of that chaos in order to try to cobble it together into some kind of comprehensive timeline.

So the biggest of 'thank you's to all those who have supported me and my feelings along the way! Whether that's my long-suffering husband and mum, who have endured every up and down, or my wider circle of family and friends, who have understood me – and my ambitions – in writing *Desperate Rants and Magic Pants*, and have contributed, promoted or advised as I've worked my way to the final version.

A special thanks to all those that contributed to the podcast *Making Babies* – particularly those who have so generously allowed me to report their stories here, which has ultimately helped make the book a more inclusive place for people to come if they want to join in the fertility conversation. I will not have represented

Acknowledgements

every experience – far from it (maybe this is a sign there are more podcast series to come). But I hope I have gone some way to widening the awareness of people's differing challenges and pathways to parenthood.

Thank you to all of those who have listened to the podcast, viewed my TEDx talk *Fertility and the Forgotten Sex* or watched my ITV documentary *Miscarriage: The Hidden Loss*. Thank you to Royal Television Society Cymru for recognising the value of that documentary and awarding it with Best Factual. I'm particularly grateful to those who were bravely interviewed for the documentary, to the producers at ITV who gently encouraged me to film, and to the wonderful Fertility Network UK, who helped me launch the podcast initially and continue to have my back with the work I have done since.

To anyone who has ever sent me correspondence or posted a social media comment expressing how my various publications or broadcasts may have helped you just a little bit on your journeys, you have no idea how much that lifted me. It was the support and encouragement I needed to keep me talking, producing and writing when I had moments of doubt and a lingering anxiety about speaking out. It was the motivation I required to push myself on to finish *Desperate Rants and Magic Pants*.

In the writing process, my sanity has also been saved many times by my editor at Y Lolfa, Carolyn Hodges, who has kept me on schedule and been invaluable in getting the book into the place it is today. Also, thanks to those who kindly read the proofs before publication and helped me feel more at ease about what I'd poured out on to paper.

My gratitude also goes out to the Books Council of Wales, without whom this would not have been possible. Such organisations ensure authors in Wales can continue to write about important, and often niche, subjects which need a voice, and which may otherwise not get that platform.

This book is all about breaking the taboos and continuing to normalise the fertility conversation. So to you, the reader, I'd just like to say: please do keep talking about these experiences rather than suffering in silence.

Andrea Byrne
September 2024

Also from Y Lolfa:

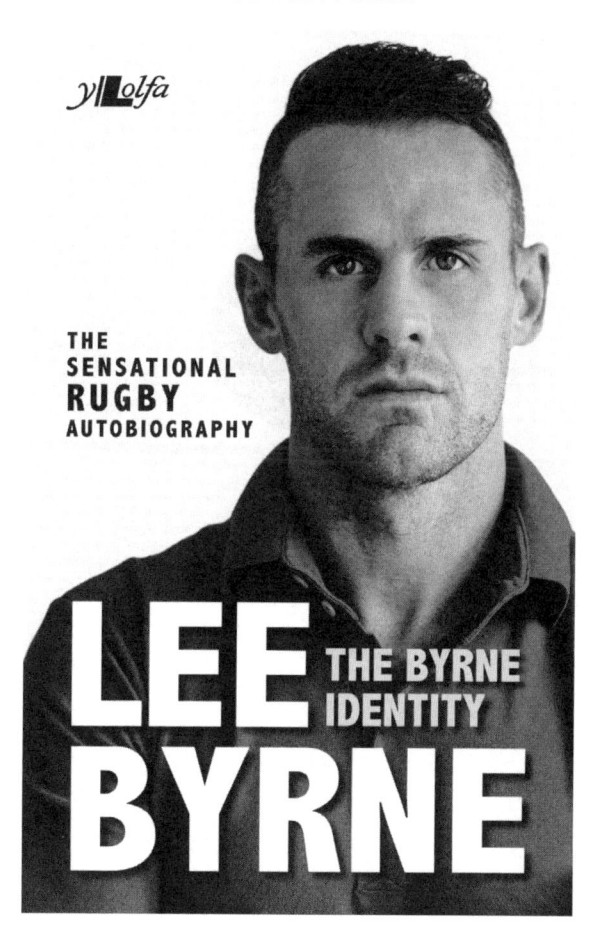

THE SENSATIONAL RUGBY AUTOBIOGRAPHY

LEE BYRNE
THE BYRNE IDENTITY

Charting his unlikely route from humble beginnings on a tough Bridgend estate and labouring on building sites to the top of world rugby as a Grand Slam winner and Test Lion, Lee Byrne's frank and powerful autobiography lifts the lid on off-field rifts and sheds new light on one of the brightest talents to grace the Welsh game.

£9.99

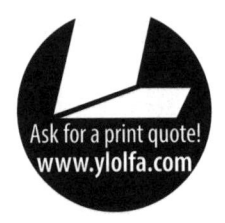